Alligator Wrestling in the Cancer Ward

Copyright © 2023 Curt Ghormley
All rights reserved.
ISBN-13: 979-8-9875884-0-6

Original cover art "The Big Leuk" by C.S. Fritz.
Author photo by Tony Weber.

Alligator Wrestling in the Cancer Ward

How a Christian Tough-Guy Survived Leukemia with Gallows Humor, One-Liners, and a Praying Posse

Curt Ghormley

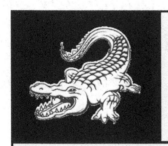

alligator
publishing
llc

www.alligatorpublishing.com

Dedication

For Kason
For Corbin
For Elizabeth

Table of Contents

Introduction..*1*

PART I: FROM FARM TO CITY...**7**

Chapter 1.. *7*
Chapter 2.. *21*
Chapter 3.. *37*
Chapter 4.. *51*
Chapter 5.. *77*

PART II: THE CANCER WARD...**111**

Chapter 6.. *111*
Chapter 7.. *129*
Chapter 8.. *159*
Chapter 9.. *177*
Chapter 10.. *195*
Chapter 11.. *211*
Chapter 12.. *235*
Afterword *243*
Acknowledgments.. *245*
About the Author.. *247*

Foreword

This is no ordinary book. But then, if you know the author, you will not expect it to be.

I became acquainted with Curt Ghormley in the early 1980s when he was a dynamic leader among the young singles at the church I pastored. We got reacquainted years later when my wife and I moved into the Benton, Kansas, neighborhood where he and Lynn have lived ever since they married in 1983.

Some of Curt's best friends (e.g., Clark and Darla, Gene and Carol) are also best friends of mine, and we are unanimous in our opinion that Curt is a very unique character. I know that's poor English, because "unique" literally means "one of a kind," so the adjective "very" is redundant. Nevertheless, it communicates something important about Curt, for he is, indeed, *very much* one of a kind.

Alligator Wrestling in the Cancer Ward is part schtick, part devotional, part psychological drama, part stream of consciousness, part confessional, and thoroughly engaging. Curt has an amazing vocabulary. In fact, I guarantee you will find words you've never seen before. That may be because they are extremely esoteric or because Curt just made them up. Others, like "throughput," are legitimate words but are given juicy new meanings you won't find in the dictionary.

No one loves the hospital, any more than the dentist's office, but Curt paints the hospital as a holy place and the caregivers as heroes and saints. I suspect none of his doctors or nurses will ever forget the tough guy who occupied that room on 7-North for three months in 2022. The dreaded C-word never faced a more formidable foe than C. Ghormley.

If you, or someone you love, are facing trauma of any sort, this book will help you process the experience. I recommend that you read it, but only a chapter at a time. In between your tears and laughter, you will find yourself wrestling also, if not with alligators, at least with yourself and your assumptions about life and death. In the unlikely event you get bogged down and are tempted to set the book aside, I urge you to *at least* read Chapter 9. My suspicion is that it will motivate you to go back to where you left off and resume your reading. There is something valuable in each chapter.

Curt does not know what the next chapter of his life looks like, but of course, none of us does. But he does know the *last* chapter because he knows the One who wrote the Book. He would clearly like for you to know Him, too.

Michael P. Andrus
Pastor, First Evangelical Free Church, Retired

Author's Note

Full disclosure: There were no alligators in the Cancer Center at Ascension St. Francis Hospital in Wichita, Kansas, in the summer of 2022; and if there had been, I would have made myself scarce, doctor's orders notwithstanding. I have never wrestled an alligator, nor have I ever had the faintest inclination to do so (I have never even noodled for catfish, although I know people who know people who have.) The closest I have ever been to an alligator is at the Denver Zoo.

But I can use my imagination, and in nightmarish visions, I can see myself thrashing dark water in a murky bog with an alligator longer than I am tall. I try to get my arms around the scaly hide while avoiding the teeth. I sense that it would be best to avoid the teeth.

Alligator Wrestling: Unexpected, unplanned, unpredictable, unfamiliar, terrifying, no rules, unlikely to end well. These words describe the experience of wrestling with cancer during my Leukemia Summer Surprise Tour in 2022.

Cancer is a subject of which I had almost zero knowledge before beginning this unexpected journey. To give context to some of the events related to this book, I have provided background on various pharmaceutical medications, surgical procedures, and hospital practices. While I have made a good-faith effort to be accurate, my accuracy may be questionable – or downright wrong in some cases. These errors are my own and are not attributable to anyone other than myself. If I have led the reader astray in drawing conclusions about this subject, I am genuinely sorry. I am no expert on anything medical, so please, let the reader beware.

Conversations and comments quoted herein are my best recollections of the words used. Still, their rendition has been massaged somewhat to make the narrative readable.

I have not knowingly compromised the intent of the speaker(s) in any case, but, on the other hand, I did not record the interchanges. Thus, I have presented them from my memory, which should not be assumed to be error-free. Again, if I have unwittingly misrepresented any claimed dialog, I apologize. I intended no harm.

During my nearly three months in the hospital, I used the Caring Bridge (CB) website to keep friends and family apprised of my status. I made journal entries every day, except for two days in intensive care when my wife and brother filled in for me. Many have asked me to publish those journal entries, and that is partly the reason for this book. The entries begin in Chapter 6 and are included at the beginning of each chapter. Notwithstanding my previous statement about re-creating certain dialog from memory, all the CB entries are exactly as originally written, the only exceptions being certain passages I have edited for clarity as when I had originally used incorrect terms for things like red blood cell counts or hemoglobin levels... which items still confuse me to this day. For publication, I corrected a few of the original mistaken entries.

Also, such a quantity of journal entries makes for tedious reading. There were stretches of many days, especially during the last month, where not much happened (besides eat, sleep, take vitals, repeat), so I omitted a few. Enough are included to keep the reader up to date with developments, but I didn't want to subject you to the drudgery of wading through all of them (It was bad enough to have to write them all in the first place.)

Scripture passages herein, unless otherwise noted, are from the New International Version as found at www.biblehub.com. Those Scriptures appearing in the Caring Bridge journal entries are King James Version, except for those few otherwise noted.

Curt Ghormley
Benton, Kansas, February 2023

Introduction

Except for the cancer, I was really in pretty good shape. If, that is, you didn't count the fatigue, labored breathing, bruising, swelling, and what might have been a canker sore.

Minor irritants, nothing more.

But then the nurse introduced me to an ER bed, stabbing the back of my hand to drip a plastic bag of goop into my arm. The emergency room doctor launched into a lecture on the differences between lymphoma and leukemia. Listening to his perplexing speech – *Why are we talking about this?* – it dawned on me that I would probably not spend the night at home. And I didn't – neither that night, nor the next 82 in a row.

He said I had leukemia. It made no sense, but the people in scrubs seemed to accept it. It was odd that they took it so calmly.

Because, that's like, cancer. Right?

After an ambulance ride with a pleasant, although unengaged EMT – this was my fight, not hers – I let the unfamiliar 12 x 14 cancer ward room soak in. As the confusion dissipated, I turned the leukemia word over in my mind. Like the tongue seeking a missing tooth, I kept wandering back to it. At length, I considered the possibility: *What if I do have leukemia? What then?*

At that point, the beginnings of a new determination slowly crept over me: *Whatever procedure or pain they must inflict on me, I will embrace it and prevail. I will accept physical discomfort with resiliency and humor.* Maybe gallows humor – there should be plenty of material close at hand – but humor, nonetheless.

It was not a resolution so much as a working hypothesis: *I'm a tough guy. In fact, I am the toughest hombre you have ever seen in a cancer ward. I am Chuck Norris. I am John Wayne, Sylvester Stallone, and Dave Bautista all rolled into one.*

At least, that was the persona I intended to project. It's not true, you understand… I'm as wimpy as the next guy, but I took it as my story and decided I would go with it.

Why would I consider making such a bold proclamation, sure to be met with cautious skepticism from strangers and dismissive eye-rolling from friends? I think it was because of the sneaking suspicion that what I really feared was the shrinking, cowering timidity that would surely arise from the question: *What will life do to me next?*

Was it merely a coping mechanism? *Probably,* I thought, *but it's my coping mechanism, so get used to it.*

There would be plenty of fear and uncertainty, but the longer I considered it that night, the more determined I became that neither would be the boss of me. *Because I'm a tough guy.* I rolled it over in my mind, testing the claim.

What brought me to that place? I had never considered that I had more physical stamina than anyone else and probably less than many. My forte had always been verbal and relational skills rather than muscular fortitude. I could run a microphone under a spotlight in front of a group with no problem. But a physical confrontation… that was not me.

Until it was. Once faced with a life-and-death requirement for actual endurance – hard, physical, gasping, grit-your-teeth endurance – I tested the notion that perhaps I was not without capability. There were events in my past that might serve me in this unknown extremity if only I could grab hold of the lessons.

*****

Sometime around my sixth-grade year, I trooped to the cafeteria with my grade school classmates, stood obediently in line for my hot lunch, and quietly took my seat at a table with other boys. With a devilish look in his eye, the kid across from me grabbed my dessert cinnamon roll as soon as I sat down. He immediately licked it, his tongue slobbering over the icing. He then licked his own cinnamon roll in the same disgusting manner, placed them both on his tray, and grinned at me.

I stared at him, aghast at the audacity, my face beginning to burn with humiliation. Then, to my everlasting disgrace, I shrugged, said nothing, and ate the remainder of my lunch in silence. He wolfed down his lunch and both cinnamon rolls. I don't remember his name.

Today, I would tip his tray into his lap and quite possibly knock him over backward in his chair. I would, of course, do that in a sincere spirit of Christian love and compassion, for I am a pleasant, mature, Scripture-loving, mild-mannered Christian who just happens to be the toughest hombre you have ever met. Or at least, who wants you to think so.

Theological Contemplations

I have concluded that toughness, the essential survival skill in a life-and-death battle with the Big L, is not incompatible with Christian virtue, but is the embodiment of such. That character trait was developed over time and was never an intended goal.

I didn't make this up on my own, and no one ever sat me down and explained why I should be tough… but as a young man, I saw it demonstrated without words by my dad. Later, I found many situations managing life and career where there was no effective substitute for showing strength. I'm sort of accustomed to living with failure — it having been such a constant companion and all — but weakness, timidity, fear, retreat: these I cannot abide.

The Apostle John writes to his "dear children" in his first epistle; specifically, he calls out young men and fathers: I write to you, fathers, because you know Him who is from the beginning. I write to you, young men, because you are strong, and the word of God lives in you, and you have overcome the evil one (1 John 2:14).

It is probably time for us to recognize that we have a responsibility to acknowledge a few things: that we can be strong, and that the Word of God has authority, and that the devil can actually be overcome; and all this because we "know Him who is from the beginning."

How is this sort of spiritually healthy toughness developed? And what does it look like?

Jacksonville Naval Air Station, 1942

My father served in the U.S. Navy from 1941 to 1946. He was from Hutchinson, Kansas, and I think the prospect of endless wheat fields year after year, the grinding poverty of the Great Depression, and a deep, abiding (yet never spoken) patriotism led him to the recruiter. The world was going to war – it was clear to him and everyone around him at the time – and he would do his duty. He enlisted in February of 1941, ten months before Pearl Harbor. During World War II, he served in an aircraft maintenance role, ultimately fueling Navy aircraft on Guam in the Mariana Islands, South Pacific.

He was 26 when he joined. He had been a farmer, truck driver, and mechanic. He shared a last name with U.S. Navy Admiral Robert L. Ghormley, then on active duty in the Pacific theatre. At best, there was only a distant relationship, but it caught the attention of officers. The name, his evident mechanical aptitude, and the fact he was a few years older than other recruits landed him a promotion to Petty Officer.

I had never thought of him as a tough guy, certainly no fighter or brawler, but (like every other boy since the world began), I was intrigued by his war stories. Such as they were.

At Jacksonville Naval Air Station, he was occasionally assigned to supervise the KP – Kitchen Police – detail. On one of these occasions, they were to mop the floor in the mess hall. Dad gave the appropriate directions and worked alongside the men.

When he asked one of the sailors to start mopping the floor, the man deliberately rested the mop in the bucket, folded his arms, looked at Dad, and offered a contemptuous smile. He had no intention of mopping the floor.

At that point, all work in the mess hall abruptly stopped. The silence was palpable as all eyes turned toward Dad.

Military discipline depends on whether a single sailor or soldier will obey a single non-commissioned officer's order. Obedience, not insubordination, must follow an order. Otherwise, discipline will evaporate; there will be no effectiveness, no work... and no clean floor in the mess hall. Unacceptable.

The sailor, very muscular and very black, was a head taller than Dad's 5' 10". Because of the heat and humidity, most men worked with shirts off, and this man's muscles bulged.

To hear Dad tell it, he squared off in front of the sailor. "Mop the floor," he said flatly.

The man returned his stare, a smirky smile on his face, and hissed through his teeth in a soundless laugh. *Why don't you make me*, was the unspoken challenge.

With a swift backhand, Dad reached up and slapped him across his massive chest. "I told you to mop the floor, sailor!" and then turned his back, resuming his own mopping.

After a few seconds' pause, the sailor slowly turned, took up his mop, and obeyed. In the mess hall, the others got back to work.

As a ten-year-old listening to this story, I was spellbound. "What would you have done if he had not followed your order?" I asked Dad.

With characteristic diffidence, Dad shrugged. "I don't know," he said. "He could have broken me in two if he wanted."

Toughness is where you find it.

My education in toughness is the substance of this book, and that education began sometime before high school.

PART I: FROM FARM TO CITY

Chapter 1

Raised on a small farm in Kansas near the Oklahoma border, I was accustomed to working from an early age. The expectation was that after school and Saturdays were for work on the farm. We didn't call it chores because that seemed a little old-fashioned. Instead, depending on the time of year, I helped by working in the fields with an elderly but reliable John Deere D-model or LA Case tractor. I mowed the grass around the outbuildings, helped herd cattle, pitched hay, and helped fix the fences. I turned mattresses, hung laundry *(woman's work!)*, tended vegetables and other necessities. Some jobs were pleasant; most were not; most involved dust or chiggers or spiders; nearly all involved sweat except the ones that involved frozen fingers and toes.

The big event of the year was the wheat harvest. Dad and I did this with a Minneapolis Moline tractor, an Allis Chalmers pull-type combine (with a tiny five-foot header), and two pickup trucks. The pickup beds were fashionably outfitted with loose gunny sacks to keep the grain from leaking out on the way to the elevator.

While Dad ran Minnie and Allis, I drove our Chevy half-ton short bed or my granddad's battered Chevy three-quarter-ton long bed to the COOP. After a couple of years of this, I actually did so legally. We did not live far from town, and virtually every farm boy in my class and many girls did the same during harvest.

I was not much for sports. An injury at age nine left me with near blindness in my left eye, and my peripheral vision on that side was virtually non-existent. Nevertheless, as one of the tallest boys in seventh grade, I met what I perceived to be society's expectations and dutifully suited up for basketball. Playing center, with no left-side vision, I was regularly clocked on the side of the head with the ball during practice.

Pre-teen boys are pretty forgiving of this sort of thing. Or not.

After a humiliating bench-warming year, I gave up on sports with a sense of relief. I was not prone to athletic endeavor; I had neither the coordination nor the instinct for it, and the physical limitation gave me an excuse to avoid it altogether. I came to see it as a blessing. The injury had steered me into much more productive paths. Such is the economy of God's workmanship.

Hence the after-school work. However, it was a tiny farm and could not keep me busy. Dad worked full-time delivering rural mail for the post office, and his route responsibilities typically gave him half-days available. After my two older brothers left home, he developed many extraordinarily creative and labor-saving mechanical solutions, for which I had approximately zero appreciation at the time: A home-brew truck on an Army surplus Dodge 6 x 6 chassis to deliver cattle feed from silo to trough; a tall, rolling A-frame with chain hoist to pull an engine; a hydraulic lift for the Minnie to add a front-end bucket. He should have been a mechanical engineer, but the Great Depression and World War II intervened in his life and times.

We do not always get to choose the trials we face; only how we face them.

Chapter 1

It has occurred to me only belatedly that perhaps he created the labor-saving solutions because his two capable sons were grown and away and no longer available, while the one left was much better suited to more sedate and indoor pursuits.

Which was why, two months after my fourteenth birthday, Mom took me to the town's grocery store and introduced me to the store owner. After a very brief conversation, he told me to show up for work the next day after school. It was news to me.

He said, "We'll be able to pay you a dollar-ten."

I struggled to make sense of the situation, but in the pregnant pause that followed, it seemed that an expression of gratitude should have been forthcoming. "Fine," I managed, perplexed. "Thank you, sir!"

I had no idea what his gibberish "dollar-ten" statement meant. This was 1968, and minimum wage was a novel concept in a farming community. Grown-ups were suspicious of it because it smacked of socialism, would no doubt lead to a Commie takeover, and soon we would all be wearing gray coveralls and working in a tractor factory. Which was why every household owned a shotgun.

While I had heard of minimum wage on the evening Huntley-Brinkley Report, the significance was lost on me. Imagine my shock and delight when I discovered I could be paid $2.20 for working a mere two hours sacking groceries after school. On Fridays, it was four hours, or $4.40, and on Saturdays, a total of six hours for $6.60. That amounted to $19.80 every week. With my first paycheck, I was suddenly seized with a full appreciation of the free market – Commie takeover or not.

The grocery store: Respectfully, work it was not. A few days before, I had been making $3.00 twice a month helping the octogenarian lady on the edge of town with her shrubs and lawn.

Somehow, the $19.80 turned into something less than $19.80 when I got the paycheck, but who cared? Nobody I knew understood how that worked or where the mysterious "deducts" went, but the leftover riches were fairly astonishing. Furthermore, sacking groceries at "a dollar-ten" was infinitely preferable to working the East 40 on an LA Case for no pay.

High school was work, school plays, band, vocal music, forensics (state speech), debate, and classes — anything that could be done without the humiliation of physical coordination. I became increasingly involved in vocal performances before an audience.

I took an event to the forensics contest in my senior year. It was held at a small college an hour's drive away. Five of us, besides the coach, traveled in the school car, a new Chevy Impala. I managed to get into the finals round, which took all day, and then we had to wait for the awards ceremony to collect my medal.

The others were predictably impatient with me because the lateness of the hour meant we would not be stopping for a take-out hamburger on the way home.

But the worst part was my double booking — that same night was the spring vocal concert. I had a solo number, and as it happened, I was the opening number in the show. We left the speech tournament 65 minutes before the concert was to start. Fortunately, the coach was a crazy woman behind the wheel, and we made the trip in record time. You gotta love a full-size Chevy with a 350 V-8.

I dashed into the auditorium, calmed my breathing for a few seconds, and reflected on whether I could remember the words to "Maria" from *West Side Story*. The arrangement we were using started with a very 1970s-dramatic "Maria!" intoned by the soloist in a dreamy, speaking voice. Then the piano sounded the opening chord, and the lyrics began.

That night, I donned my school blazer, stepped onto the stage in front of the assembled choir, watched the curtain part, noted the shadowy figures of the crowd of assembled townspeople, and thought to myself, *what was that girl's name??*

But I figured it out and acted as though the long pause was merely to let the anticipation build.

Vocal music was not the only highlight. As a sophomore, our band director moved me from cornet to tuba, probably because the first chair trumpet player was much better than I. While I had some modicum of talent, I would never be able to compete with him. I fell in love with the tuba. The school purchased four brand new Miraphone brass tubas: Four-valve, rotary-valve instruments.

These were not the white fiberglass sousaphones you see in marching bands; these were heavy, high-quality concert horns held upright in your lap while seated. The rotary valves meant that levers operated the keys, like a French Horn, rather than pistons, like a trumpet. The purists tell me the rotary action is not quite as fast as the piston, but who cares: The cool factor of the rotary was huge. I called it lever-action. Each tuba was the price of a modest car.

Our band director was a legend in Kansas public school bands with 21 consecutive first-division ratings at state music contests. In my senior year, he announced, "Our outstanding seniors are going to play solos in our spring concerts."

It is significant, I learned, to pay attention to syntax. The word used was "concerts," not "concert." I did not yet know the Apostle Paul's analysis of Abraham's progeny in the third chapter of Galatians. He asserts that God's promise was *not* "and to his seeds," but rather, "and to his seed." Singular versus plural; it's an important distinction.

The other "outstanding seniors" played solo numbers on the big community-wide evening concert — a notable annual cultural affair in a small town. I was relegated to performing "Tubby the Tuba" at the daytime children's concert at the elementary school. I suppose these are the events that build character.

Not to minimize the technical difficulty, but Tubby the Tuba was *hard*. However, the storyline is light-hearted: Tubby feels left out and discouraged until some event makes him a hero to the band… a common theme, like Rudolph and his reindeers. Nevertheless, the technical musicality required was quite advanced.

This hill was too tall for me to climb, which is precisely why the director, a World War II fighter pilot, assigned it to me. He had flown a P-47 Thunderbolt; eight wing-mounted .50-caliber machine guns, raining death and destruction on Nazi troop trains. It took me several years to appreciate the enormous privilege of being associated with him. He stood five-foot-six with his shoes on and was a giant among men. He had a take-no-prisoners approach to discipline, and yet was approachable, gentle, entertaining, and superbly demanding. At high school reunions, we still echo his unique commands: *If I tell you to put the horn in your ear and blow, you put the horn in your ear and blow!*

Our principal saxophone player was so nervous at one state contest that she refused to play her solo. She was in the warm-up room and the judges were waiting for her next door. The director found her among well-meaning friends who consoled her as she wept. In predictably outrageous fashion, he confronted her: "Listen, I know you are upset and nervous, but music is to be made for others, not just yourself. Now dry your tears, get off your butt, get in there and play your solo!"

She wailed and then did as he said.

Our respect for him was off the chart.

Chapter 1

But in that senior year, I still had to get Tubby the Tuba under my fingers, plus a selection of other technically challenging pieces for the spring contest.

Therefore, I saw it as an incredible stroke of luck when the grocery store burned down.

During church on a Sunday morning in January, two hundred of us United Methodists heard the fire siren begin to wail.

Living in a small town, we had a volunteer fire department. A dignified local merchant, dressed in his Sunday suit, was an usher in that service. When the siren sounded as the offering was being collected, he suddenly thrust the half-filled plate of money toward a surprised parishioner and sprinted down the aisle for the front door.

Pretty cool to see that!

The place where I had worked for the last three years was a total loss. Along with half the town, I watched the smoldering structure from a block away and slowly realized I would not have a job come Monday.

As a result, that spring semester, I made a habit of staying at school for two hours after classes each day, by myself, in a band practice room. Nobody told me to, but it was either practice the tuba or watch *Star Trek* re-runs, and that seemed a little short-sighted. So, while my peers ran the basketball court in grueling practices, I ran scales, intervals, and equally grueling sixteenth-note rips on a Miraphone lever-action tuba. I learned to double-tongue and triple-tongue. I developed tone quality and disciplined breathing.

By concert time, I was ready, and Tubby never knew what hit him. I nailed him to the wall in front of 50 spellbound third graders. Success never tasted sweeter.

My other great love in high school was debate. It was for me an entertaining diversion. I came to relish the mental gymnastics of flipping from affirmative to negative: One side of the question to the other, effortlessly, with rapier-like wit, and seemingly with full conviction.

My senior year, the topic was, *Resolved: That the federal government should establish, finance, and administer programs to control air and/or water pollution in the United States.* My partner was Marge, a girl a year behind me in school with a clever mind and a winning personality. Marge and I were good in a small school but sensed we could not keep up with the fast movers from the big cities: Wichita, Topeka, Lawrence, Kansas City. So we convinced our coach (the crazy woman who drove school vehicles filled with innocent children far too fast) to let us try an alternate strategy.

In a high school debate, the usual practice is to represent either the affirmative side (in support of the resolution) or the negative side (opposed to the resolution).

In a conventional format, the affirmative team cites a plethora of evidence showing that the current system is broken and offers "Our Plan" to fix it. The negative team cites a different plethora of evidence asserting that the status quo is *not* broken, and the problems are not nearly as significant as their worthy though misguided opponents have claimed. Furthermore, "Your Plan" is illogical, unworkable, unnecessary, and probably economically disruptive.

That's how it's supposed to go, and both affirmative and negative debaters know it. We know they know it because they will switch sides after every round in a tournament (usually six in a day). An hour prior, I was on the affirmative side, but now I'm on the negative. This is actually a great way to develop critical thinking skills in teenagers.

So, we convinced the crazy driver coach to let us do something almost unheard of but legal in Kansas high school debates. We offered a "comparative-advantage" format on the negative side of the resolution. Diabolically, the format change is announced only after the round of debate has begun; it is somewhat risky, it is a nasty surprise, and it can completely disorient the affirmative team. *Perfect!*

This is comparable to the special-teams punter suddenly throwing a pass on fourth down.

Chapter 1

In the comparative-advantage approach, the negative, shockingly, agrees with the first affirmative speaker: Yes, they assert, the status quo needs to be fixed, but you have failed to show how bad the situation (in this case, environmental pollution) actually is. Furthermore, we have the plan to fix this egregious problem, and by comparison with your plan, ours offers significant advantages. Comparative-advantage.

But there is a risk with this strategy. While we are all conversant with the affirmative team's evidence, the negative team only hears the affirmative's plan halfway through the debate. If both plans are identical, the negative team is toast. They must modify their own plan on the fly, which we had to do a few times, and which, as a cerebral exercise, was a shot of adrenaline.

Marge and I were dramatically successful with this deliciously cruel, underhanded, and perfectly legal strategy.

One of the last tournaments of the year was a two-day event with scores of schools invited. The rules required four-person teams, meaning that two of us would always debate affirmative in every round and the other two negative. The effect was that the contestants were highly proficient with their evidence, and the quality of their arguments was substantially heightened.

Our comparative-advantage plan on the negative side was a killer: Marge and I went 11-1 in the 12-round tournament.

Unfortunately, our counterparts, younger and less experienced, went 1-11. Our combined team thus scored an overall record of 12-12 – no medals for us.

But what a ride that was. Marge and I had faced some of the best minds in Kansas high schools and skunked them. We did it with brains and strategy rather than brawn. As a confidence builder, nothing could have been better. Tubby should have been there, but he was still nailed to the wall in the elementary school gym. I was sure that girl with the elusive Maria name had fallen deeper in love with me.

Thus, I grew from Casper Milquetoast in sixth grade to a commanding force in high school debate, forensics, and vocal and instrumental music. All that, plus I had a job and money in the bank. I had been toughened by farm work, lonely hours in a practice room working Tubby over, and the urgent mental and verbal gymnastics of real-time debate. So yes, I grew in toughness and capability.

Nevertheless, I was unsettled inside as I contemplated college; I was deeply insecure. Despite past successes, the road ahead was uncertain and filled with likely failure.

I was determined to meet this new experience with such strength as I could muster, but I suspected that it would be inadequate for the challenge. With age, I have come to understand that the haughty, arrogant, and cynical teenager I became was a coping mechanism to free myself from, or at least conceal, my insecurity.

I did not yet know Peter's second epistle: *Promising them freedom, they themselves became slaves to corruption.* On what I hoped was the plus side, I was headed for a big university, where new experiences awaited. I had little idea what to expect and found much more than I had bargained for.

Theological Contemplations

A Christian perspective (or, as I like to think of it, the only rational perspective of a thinking man) asks whether this focus on toughness is virtue or vice. Critics generally point out that Jesus said to turn the other cheek. Wasn't he "gentle Jesus, meek and mild," after all? What about warnings against pride, which we are told "goes before destruction" and is to be avoided?

Chapter 1

First, I would say that a simple analysis of Matthew 5:39 is helpful. *But I tell you, do not resist an evil person. If anyone slaps you on the right cheek, turn to them the other cheek also.* Understanding the context should rid one of acquiescing to a defenseless fistfight. The world is predominately right-handed. Receiving a blow to your right cheek, therefore, requires your assailant to be either left-handed (an unlikely antecedent to Jesus' general instruction) or, more likely, to have used the back of his hand. The back of the hand is an insult, not a severe blow, and this Gospel passage is all in the context of suffering persecution for the supposed crime of identifying with Jesus and His people.

The lesson is that when one is persecuted for being Christian, expect it, embrace it, struggle not against it.

Conversely, when one is mugged on the street or his house is invaded, and life or dignity is threatened, he is free to meet force with force.

Second, the phrase "gentle Jesus, meek and mild" is from Charles Wesley's collection of hymns for children in 1742, not directly from the Scripture. Jesus indeed said He was meek, and in the Beatitudes (specifically Matthew 5:5), He promises His followers that "the meek shall inherit the earth." Commentators generally agree the word "meek" refers to the same concept as that of a horse under the control of its master. Strength under control means that the "meek" person has nothing to prove. New Testament meekness is such strength, and so illustrates the wisdom of Proverbs 16:32, *Better a patient person than a warrior, one with self-control than one who takes a city.*

Third, this Jesus, who described Himself as "meek and lowly in heart" in Matthew 11:29 also said He would overthrow Chorazin, Bethsaida, Tyre, and Sidon. He promised they would be brought down lower than Sodom because of their sins. As far as meekness goes, this claim was not remotely akin to weakness.

C. S. Lewis wrote of Aslan, the Christ character in *The Lion, The Witch and The Wardrobe* (Macmillan Publishing, 1950), "It's not as though he's a *tame* lion."

Jacksonville Naval Air Station, 1943

Newly promoted Chief Petty Officer Robert C. Ghormley led a hundred men as they were to be carried by bus to some activity. As ordered, the men showed up before dawn at an empty hanger to await the transportation, which, not surprisingly, was late, by several hours, as it turned out.

With nothing to do and no chow, men began to complain. Arguments ensued; trouble was brewing: Idle hands and all that.

Dad was what is called a "Chief Petty Officer (temporary)." This was a war-time rating when the demand for Chiefs far exceeded the available supply. He was permanently rated a Petty Officer First Class, but was breveted to Chief, with full responsibilities and duties of a Chief, for the duration of hostilities.

(In the same way, George Armstrong Custer, U.S. Army, was breveted to Brigadier General during the Civil War; he was later commissioned Lieutenant Colonel, regular Army, in time for his ill-fated run-in with Sitting Bull at Little Big Horn.)

There was one other Chief in the hangar that morning, and the two NCOs (non-commissioned officers) discussed the situation. They had noticed the runway near the hanger was littered with remnants of what could only have been a crashed airplane: Bits of aluminum, rubber, steel components, nuts and bolts, clumps of wiring harness, broken shards of plexiglass. The big pieces of the airframe had been removed, but the runway was trashed and unsafe. No doubt there were plans somewhere to return with a work detail or a street sweeper, but this was the Navy... and there was no telling what was up.

Dad ordered the men to fall in. Once formed, he told them they were going to sweep the runway. He and the other Chief passed out brooms, buckets and shovels from the hanger's extensive tool room, and all hands fell to the task.

Almost all hands. A cluster of three young Petty Officers stood at the edge of the pavement, watching, not working. Dad approached the group.

"What's your story, men?" he asked.

"Oh, we're Petty Officers First Class," said one, as though this were a perfectly rational explanation for their lack of involvement.

"Really," said Dad, in a reasonable tone of voice. "I'm a Chief. Get a broom."

They did.

*****

The Apostle Paul's second letter to Timothy includes this assertion: *For the Spirit God gave us does not make us timid, but gives us power, love and self-discipline (2 Timothy 1:7).*

In this sense, the tough-guy image embodies meekness (strength under control), allows unselfconscious love to flow through one as a channel of God's grace, and evidences the self-discipline to truthfully acknowledge physical and spiritual challenges and meet them head-on.

So yeah, I'm a tough guy. Tell everyone you know.

Chapter 2

I had visited the university with my parents, so I at least knew where it was and could find my dormitory, the administration building, and the fieldhouse. When it was time to make the four-hour trip to start the fall semester, I drove myself, my Mini Cooper "S" filled to window level with required college stuff.

It was a bright, beautiful summer morning, and the Mini and I made it about 12 miles before the engine died. I coasted to a stop off the road at a wide intersection, out of traffic, and there we sat. Dad was on the mail route; Mom was at work; cell phones were 15 years away, and I was left with a roadside problem.

On the farm, automotive mechanics had been a daily part of life. As much as anything, this was due to the post office mileage reimbursement policy. Dad squeezed many miles out of his mail-route car by doing the maintenance himself and retaining the income.

Unable to dodge this aspect of rural American self-sufficiency, I regularly performed oil changes and packed wheel bearings. I also changed spark plugs, gapped valves, and rotated tires. Every self-respecting farm boy, and many of the city kids, could do routine maintenance in the days before you could run the car a hundred thousand miles virtually without lifting the hood.

But when it came down to it, I had no idea why the engine had died. It was sudden and complete. I listened to the engine tick as it cooled down on a summer's day with a customary gentle Kansas breeze (15 knots with gusts to 25).

My analytical skills were limited but not non-existent. There had been no sputter, so it was not a fuel problem. Instead, it was as though someone had turned off the ignition key. I examined the key carefully and hopefully, but no, it had not flipped itself off.

What had Dad said? "If it won't run, Mister, it's either fuel or ignition. There are not any other choices."

Okay... so if it was not fuel, it was not out of gas. It was not a clogged fuel or air filter; it was not a fuel pump; it was not (thankfully) a carburetor problem; it was not a road hazard that had ripped a gasoline line. That meant ignition: Distributor cap, rotor, breaker points, coil... or broken wiring.

Broken wiring can be really hard to find.

I got out, raised the hood and stared, uncomprehending, at the tiny 1275 cc power plant. In a 1966 Mini, the engine was mounted transverse, left-to-right, rather than fore-and-aft as in, say, a Mercury Cougar V-8 that I wanted so badly I could taste it. Sort of cream yellow with narrow racing stripes, vinyl top, chocolate leather interior, 8-track tape deck, factory air conditioning, four-on-the-floor... but I digress. The Mini used this unique engine configuration to save space, given the tiny body, and because it simplified the engineering for front-wheel drive.

The sideways mount meant the four spark plugs were visible in a line across the front with big fat plug wires running to the distributor behind the faux chrome grill. The coil had a spring-loaded solenoid, making it child's play to start the car without a key (only be careful not to leave it in gear and run over yourself). It sat adjacent to the distributor and was connected to the distributor cap by a single heavy black rubber-coated wire. There was also a smaller 18-gauge insulated wire... which today was hanging loose in the Kansas breeze, frayed copper strands exposed. It drooped near a small, shiny electrical connector on the distributor with nothing attached.

Is that normal? Who knows?

With nothing else to try, I got a pair of pliers (in our household, required equipment in every vehicle) and crimped the bare wires to the empty connector. Nothing smoked (a sure harbinger of trouble to come), so I tried the ignition.

It worked. I started the engine, dropped the hood, and resumed the trip, swelling with pride and a sense that I could conquer any difficulty.

A broken primary coil wire is probably the simplest possible problem that could ever occur in a 1966 Mini Cooper (Try replacing the radiator hose, for example. It was specially manufactured with three ends; I kid you not. The space was so tight you could either see the hose clamps or touch them, but not at the same time.)

As far as conquering all difficulties, however, my farm boy innards were unsettled; I was, after all, merely one of about 5,000 incoming freshmen at a state university. Moreover, I had minimal study skills because I had not needed to work at school before. I still needed to decide what classes to take; I had no genuine interest in any major. At some level, I recognized this meant that I was headed for aimless, unsuccessful drifting in the following months and a nascent conviction that this may not end well.

I had not yet heard the aphorism, "Aim at nothing, and you will hit it every time." But I sensed trouble coming, despite the coil wire fix, and began to feel my confidence slipping away.

*****

Enrollment was a nightmare in a multi-level fieldhouse. Standing to one side of a large passageway with hundreds of fellow students flowing past, I opened the newsprint catalog to determine which courses I could take. There was a vast array of LA&S (Liberal Arts & Science) offerings. How many hours was each? What was the schedule? What was the total I could or should enroll in? If the class did not work, could I withdraw?

I found a likely suspect class, studied the included map to determine where that table was, and fought through the mass of confused undergraduate humanity only to find the class already filled.

Back to the catalog, find a second choice. Or third. Or fourth. Study the map, push my way to the table, and pull a class card.

Remember, this was 1971. The transistor itself (the basic building block of the Information Revolution) was only 15 years old. A computer was an enormous, expensive installation that took up most of the floor in the Computer Science building and, by today's standards, had almost no processing power. The widespread availability of TCP/IP, the protocol on which the internet runs, was a quarter century in the future. Everything was on paper records.

One had to possess an IBM punch card to enroll in a particular class. The number of punch cards available for each class reflected the class size. For example, large freshman mandatory classes (biology, chemistry, astronomy, etc.) were held in large lecture halls with a capacity of 200. Smaller classes (philosophy, French, English Lit, algebra) would have maybe 25.

One had to find the table for the desired class, pull a card, if available, and verify the days and times offered by the class section, and then identify another offering and repeat the process until the schedule was complete. Hopefully, it would include classes that would contribute to a bachelor's degree in an acceptable field. It was only LA&S, after all. To a non-technical farm boy, one major was pretty much like any another.

At last, I had cards for the four or five classes I had chosen. I presented them to the scheduling Nazi at the exit, and then ran the gauntlet where every student organization known to mankind recruited unsuspecting freshmen to their extracurricular groups. Environmentalists, politicos, Christians, Buddhists, gays, vegetarians, scuba divers, anti-war doves, ROTC recruiters, free marketers, sportsmen, Spanish speakers, rock climbers, Greek houses... sheesh! Who has time to go to school?

Chapter 2

Buying textbooks was approximately the same routine but in a much tighter venue at the University Bookstore. Bringing the books back to the dorm room, I stacked them on my desk, regarded them skeptically, and suspected I would never read most of them. Turns out I was right, and I have the grades to prove it.

*****

Making new friends was more challenging than one might have thought. To my dismay, not one of the 160 men in that dormitory knew of my earlier high school debate record. No one cared that I remembered Maria's name just in time or that I had seriously given Tubby the business in a practice room. I met a few guys in passing and virtually no girls... it's hard to develop an effective pickup line in a lecture class of 200 when every other freshman guy is attempting exactly the same thing.

The one bright spot, and it eventually became a life-changer, was an upperclassman down the hall who befriended me. We would sit in his room and talk philosophy – sort of. I became aware that every conversation turned to church, religion, the Bible, Jesus. But he was affable, friendly, and seemed normal. In November, he invited me to a rally at a local church on a Friday evening.

Now, I drove a Mini Cooper; I subscribed to *Road & Track* magazine, and I fancied myself something of a sports car aficionado. In my world, a rally meant an open-air parking lot competition with orange plastic cones. Drivers would maneuver their Fiats, MGs, Austins, Triumphs, or BMWs through the course for the best time. So when he invited me, I thought, *Yeah, cool,* and accepted his invitation. He himself drove a 1965 Plymouth the size of a tank, with handling and fuel economy to match, but I figured it was just a school car. Maybe the church had a lighted parking lot, seeing this was a Friday night event.

Imagine my surprise.

There were about 50 of us in the church basement. Some were upperclassmen; some were apparent freshmen like me. We sat classroom-style in folding chairs; a piano struck a chord, we all rose to our feet, and the assembled crowd sang hymns with raucous abandon. The people were smiling, polite, energetic, and appeared to be quite genuine. There was nothing campy or cynical about it. Despite suspicions, I found myself enjoying the group.

There was something wholesome and fun about the proceeding.

We sang a few hymns I had never heard before, but I could sight-read the music and surely impressed those around me with my confident bass line. At length, we took our seats and an old man, maybe 35, approached the podium. He was a retired Canadian hockey player who opened a massive black Bible and began to tell stories of hockey exploits. I took this to be the "put the audience at ease" part, and it was. Soon he launched into a personal account of how his life had spiraled downward morally and spiritually as his hockey career had flourished.

He quoted a few Bible verses and described a personal encounter with Jesus. It appeared he was speaking of a spiritual, non-visible encounter that had occurred as he prayed rather than a physical apparition or miraculous meeting. Once I understood this, I felt more at ease. He then talked about how life had improved after meeting Jesus. Eventually, he left hockey and took a position with a not-for-profit Christian organization so that he could… have meetings like this one.

I was not widely experienced, but I recognized what he was selling. This was the Christian gospel in four easy points: God loves you, you're a sinner, Jesus will forgive your sins, and you should pray the Sinner's Prayer.

It was good that I had heard it all before and was firmly in Jesus' camp. I had been to church all my life, was a regular attender, and had gone on all the youth group summer trips. As he spoke, I tried to recall the specific time I had verbalized faith in Christ; I came up blank. I was sure I had done so… or maybe I never had.

Doubts began. Making that decision is not the sort of thing you write down, except I found out later that it was *precisely* the sort of thing you write down.

Before he got to the juicy part, I had my story straight in my head: I would claim that I had accepted Christ at an earlier age, had tried to read the Bible and live for Him, but that now on this night, I was going to pray whatever he recommended as sort of a reaffirmation. This internal narrative allowed me to deal with my cognitive dissonance. While I knew the facts of the Gospel, I had never acted on it. I was bugged by the notion that it had been meaningless to me on those very few occasions when I had tried to read the Bible. It was like reading someone else's mail.

Sure enough, he led in group prayer. I prayed silently, repeating his words: *Lord, I know I'm a sinner. Tonight, I ask you to forgive my sin, come into my heart, and make my life new. Amen.*

It was not an emotional event for me, but at the hockey guy's suggestion, I told the Plymouth guy about it. He seemed impressed and happy, and I thought, *Of course, you are — you got a live one tonight.* I had no idea of the changes about to take place in my thoughts and priorities.

Classes were not forgotten, but over the next few days, I found myself reading a borrowed Bible at every opportunity. The Gospel of Matthew seemed like a logical place to start, being the first one in the right half of the book. I met with the Plymouth guy several times, and he suggested I memorize some Scripture verses.

Say what?

At first repulsed by the idea, I took one of his little sub-wallet size cards and learned Galatians 2:20 because I did not want to offend him. *I have been crucified with Christ; it is no longer I who live but Christ who lives in me. The life I now live in the flesh I live by faith in the Son of God, who loved me and gave himself for me.*

The more I thought about that passage, the more I craved to know.

In what way have I been crucified? Because last I checked, I have not been nailed to a cross. How is it that Christ lives in me? What does that even mean? How is it that I live life in the flesh by faith? And why would he give himself for me? *What's wrong with me?* I thought. *Am I now a Jesus freak?*

Maybe so, but I found myself not caring. I was consumed with the Bible. After Matthew, I skipped Mark and Luke because I figured they were the same story again (*Wrong!*), but I read John, Acts, Romans, the Corinthians, and more. I understood only pieces of it and sensed strongly that most of the message went right past me, but I was unstoppable. The University Bookstore had Bibles in the Religion section. I bought a hardback Revised Standard Version of "The Bible" (not the "Holy Bible," you understand, this being higher education) for $1.35.

Plymouth invited me to a men's Bible study and gave me a paperback workbook. I filled it out scrupulously: Lots of Q&A, lots of going back and forth answering, *What's this verse say? How is this passage different from that passage?* I recognized the writer wanted me to become familiar with the Book, mainly the New Testament, and I dived right in.

A sidelight to this conversion experience – for that is precisely what it was, although I did not have the word for it at the time – occurred a month later, over Christmas break, back home on the farm. One night, I went to a party at a friend's place: High school friends, the old crowd.

You must understand I had never tasted alcohol before. It was not used in our family, and I had never run with a crowd that drank.

Chapter 2

But there were plenty of suds at this party; I was nearly eighteen and curious about what being drunk would feel like. Of course, I knew this was wrong for a Christian — *be not drunk with wine,* and all that. But I rationalized that the Holy Spirit was working in me, changing my desires and habits. By the time Spring Break rolled around, I would be a much more mature Christian and probably would not *want* to get drunk. Besides that, I had learned that Plymouth kept a close eye on his new converts in the dorm to keep us on the straight and narrow, and I did not want to suffer the humiliation of a rebuke.

The obvious conclusion was that if I were going to get drunk, the time was now, and the place was here. I started chugging wine. It was red.

I have only a vague recollection of Wesley driving me home in my car around midnight. There must have been another car following to take him back to the party. The next morning, I found my cast-off clothes in unusual places; I slept late and had a throbbing headache and a dry mouth. To their credit, my parents did not confront me about it, although I am sure they knew what was up.

The loss of control I experienced that night was fundamentally unsettling. I resolved never to do it again, and I never did.

In the spring semester, I took a job in the dormitory cafeteria — minimum wage was now $1.60, *woohoo!* — and plunged into more Bible study. Classes too, but my first love was Bible. I began to memorize the Topical Memory System, 60 verses on various topics, published by The Navigators. Walking to class across campus found me with a tiny vinyl verse pack in hand, flipping through Scriptures and reciting them out loud to ensure word-perfect memory. Other students looked sideways at me, but I didn't care.

I still know all the verses, with references.

The rest of college was full of classes, homework, evening Bible studies, and cafeteria work. I was promoted to Line Captain, in charge of student help, for a five-cent per hour raise, then Senior Line Captain for another ten cents, and ultimately to Clerk-Typist for yet another 30 cents. Righteous money at $2.05 an hour.

I majored, finally, in Speech Communication with a double major in Personnel Administration, which we now call Human Resources. I found it boring then and boring now, but I'm happy some people like that sort of thing. By the time my senior year rolled around, we had 40 men from our dormitory – 25% of the population – in regular weekly Bible studies.

When I graduated, I chose to stay in the college town and work a blue-collar job for a year.

Dad had been blue-collar all his life, although he had two years of business college – a considerable accomplishment for a man completely without assets who had turned 18 during the Great Depression. Nevertheless, he usually found himself doing the work rather than supervising those who did. The Chief Petty Officer role was probably the professional highlight of his life. Five years after his discharge, he scratched out bare subsistence during the worst drought of the century on a Kansas farm with a wife and two boys.

Both my older brothers had served in the military during the Vietnam era, one Air Force and one Navy. In my mind, they had been there and done that; I had not.

I could see that my career path would take me directly from college to a white-collar job, probably in sales and an environment where a suit and tie were required. I would never have had the experience of working on the factory floor and being "one of the guys." Was that important? It seemed like it at the time. Call it bragging rights; call it street cred. I wanted some, and I had none.

So, one summer morning after college, I donned jeans, work boots, and a clean tee shirt. I walked the industrial section of that university town, applying for a job at every business I passed. By 2:00 p.m., I had secured a position as a spray painter at a small steel fabrication plant. I worked there for 18 months – minimum wage was now $3.25! – and then moved to the big city to see what might be next.

Theological Contemplations

On the check-in desk at the dormitory cafeteria entrance, someone had graffitied, "Curt loves Jesus." Another wit came along and added, "So do I." A third scribbled, "You should too."

I learned some things working with students.

One, I wasn't very good at it. I tend to be simultaneously overbearing and apologetic, which is a neat trick if you can pull it off, seeing these are at opposite ends of the relationship spectrum. I can come off as both rude and spineless, not ideal traits for an emissary of the Gospel. But it doesn't keep me from banging away at it. Taking my cue from that eminent philosopher Dirty Harry, "A man's got to know his limitations," I try to guard against both extremes.

Two, while many converts confess faith in Jesus for the forgiveness of sins, it is unusual to trip across one who can communicate that message to others. Less common yet is the one who can train someone else to do the same. This requires not only knowledge of the subject but also time... a great deal of time, not to mention the willingness to be disappointed.

Three, most of us clods stumbling through life need practical helps to manage the Christian life. We need simple recipes for studying the Bible, for sharing our faith, or even for an effective Bible reading program. Simple is good.

Most of us who call ourselves Christians struggle with staying the course. It was not easy being a born-again Christian at a godless state university in the 1970s. While there were some natural antagonists (a particular Western Civ professor comes to mind, the toad), I admit that at that time, I took myself far too seriously. I felt an internal compulsion to practice the faith. I was so hopeful of influencing others to do the same that any degree of failure to do so felt like... failure.

So why not bag it and go back to chasing girls? For one, I wasn't any good at that either, and for two... I had made a commitment. The question was then, and still is now, whether I would remain true to that commitment.

My high school peer group in the 1970s (much like high school peer groups today and in every other generation) found it entertaining to have erudite philosophical discussions. We tried to identify and solve the world's problems. As I participated in these bull sessions, it occurred to me that life was filled with unrelated and contradictory purposes, reflected in popular wisdom, such as:

- Study hard and be a model student, or
- Ignore school and get a job as a plumber or electrician or mechanic, or
- Be moral, raise a family and be a pillar of the community, or
- Live a solitary life minding your own business, or
- Throw away outdated morals and live for the moment, regardless of consequences.

Chapter 2

And so on. As a child, sleeping in an upstairs bedroom in a drafty old farmhouse, I loved the heavy quilt cover Mom put on my bed. It was old and tattered and featured multiple designs and floral squares, but it trapped body heat and kept me warm. The designs intrigued me, as they all appeared to be different. In my teen years, I considered that our discussions of the variegated aims of life were similarly differentiated. I wondered what common thread could hold together such disparate views of life.

Fast-forward to my freshman year in college as a new Christian. With my new-found faith, I had the quite naïve conviction that I could unlock all the wisdom yet hidden from the great unwashed masses of unenlightened knaves. Yet, I still contemplated that quilt work, representing all those differing philosophies. So it was that when I came across Colossians 1:17, I was struck by the simplicity of the passage and the centrality of Christ that Paul proclaimed: *He is before all things, and in Him all things hold together.*

In Jesus Christ, I realized, all the issues of life find their definition. I reasoned that if that were the case, it was only right and proper for me to make Him the center of my hopes, dreams, pursuits, and lifestyle. Peter said, *Lord, to whom shall we go? You have the words of eternal life. (John 6:68)* I committed to that truth in a quiet dormitory room in the spring of 1972. To be sure, it was then, and is now, aspirational rather than descriptive. But there it is.

Someone said committing oneself to the Lordship of Christ is "One big Yes, and a bunch of little Uh-Huhs."

That time in my dorm was one big "Yes." Since then, the infinite series of little "Uh-Huhs" have been merely a matter of remaining consistent with that first decision. I have failed and deviated more than I have succeeded and stayed true. God forgives and restores.

Dunkirk, 1940

In the early and very dark days of World War II, before the U.S. entered the war, there occurred a poignant scene for Great Britain and her Allies. Some 350,000 Allied troops, the bulk of the effective fighting force, were stranded literally at the edge of the sea at Dunkirk, a coastal city in northern France. The enemy German offensive, with better equipment and many more troops, had pushed the Allies to retreat. They were ready to either shell them to pieces or accept their unconditional surrender.

A senior British officer, committed to a suicidal rear-guard action to hold the line, sent a message to his commander in England pleading for rescue across the English Channel. He included the simple three-word phrase, "But if not."

It makes little sense to modern ears, safe in 21st-century America. In 1940, however, virtually every Westerner was familiar with the King James Bible, and many immediately understood the reference to Daniel 3:18. Shadrach, Meshach, and Abednego had been brought before King Nebuchadnezzar and were challenged to worship the statue of the King. Otherwise, they would be cast into "the burning fiery furnace." They refused to do so, being worshippers of God alone; they asserted that their God could deliver them from the furnace. But even if He did not bring such deliverance, they still had no intention of bending to Nebuchadnezzar's will: "But if not..."

In 1940, the meaning was clear: You either rescue us very soon, or we will die fighting.

Was this excessive pride or something noble? In this context, it was not pride but humility. The field commander had committed himself and his men to the service of his king; he was determined to carry out his commitment to a power higher than himself. In that sense, he was merely an instrument obedient to the king's authority. One greater than he was part of the story.

Chapter 2

For the record, the sealift that carried out the successful evacuation of the army from Dunkirk has become the stuff of legend. Navy ships, civilian yachts, privately owned fishing boats, basically anything with a motor that could float all responded. There was immediate, patriotic, and selfless fervor to bring as many soldiers across the Channel as possible. In all, about 338,000 were rescued.

*****

I take great motivation from the story of Gideon and his 300 warriors chasing the kings of Midian (Judges 8:4). Gideon and his boys, in a foot chase of many hours' duration, crossed the River Jordan, worn out and hungry. But they were not dispirited: *Faint, yet pursuing,* says the record.

I challenge myself: I know you're faint, but are you still pursuing? Are you going to deviate from the path or not? Are you going to set a course and then suddenly waffle on the direction? To be sure, some obstructions loom large in the road ahead. The fact is that big decisions in the Christian life, rather than bringing one's progress to a stop at those obstacles, serve to guide one *through* those obstacles. This is true when one hears bad news regarding money, marriage, child-rearing, career, or anything else threatening one's faith.

Even including a cancer diagnosis.

Chapter 3

Kansas City beckoned opportunity in the summer of 1977. Knowing it was time to get on with my life and try to find a career, I called a friend who lived in the city in a two-bedroom apartment with three other guys, all Christians I had known in college. They invited me to crash in the living room; one of them was moving out in a few weeks, and I would be able to take his place. My share of the rent was affordable, even though I had little savings.

I moved in and took my rotation with house cleaning and cooking. Days were spent with a fifty-cent newspaper from a dispenser at the clubhouse scouring the Help Wanted ads, making calls, and driving to interviews. I ran back and forth across Johnson County, Wyandotte County, and Jackson County, putting my best foot forward.

At first, I was selective, scratching some jobs off the list if they seemed unattractive. I was looking for business-to-business sales and the respectability I thought it would entail. But, after a month, I became open-minded in inverse proportion to my dwindling funds. At length, I took a sales position selling industrial maintenance supplies... roof patch and asphalt patch.

It paid $3.50 an hour (25 cents above minimum wage!), and the sales manager did not want to hire me. He explained that single men with college degrees were unpredictable and that I would probably quit for a better job at higher pay at the first opportunity.

I suggested that (a) he might solve that problem by paying substantially better, and (b) I had a bachelor's degree in Personnel Administration and was well acquainted with federal and state statutes that made that sort of discrimination patently illegal and actionable in a court of law. (That may have stretched my expertise just a tad, but only one of us knew that.)

He swallowed hard and hired me on the spot. It was perhaps not the best way to begin a working relationship, but I was becoming desperate and needed money coming in instead of going out.

It was a terrible job. There was virtually no training and no company support. The office experience was a miserable bullpen with four of us at tiny desks, each with a telephone and a Yellow Pages, our prospect list. I resolved to stay out of the office as much as possible. I spent my days in my Chevy Vega, cold-calling uninterested plant supervisors with uninteresting asphalt products.

Just as the sales manager had predicted, I continued to chase other positions. I figured it was his own fault.

At some point, I was given a list of the twenty largest employers in the Kansas City metropolitan area and the suggestion to send them each a resume. Brilliant, I know; probably no one had ever thought of that before. So, I spent my last $300.00 (*Three hundred dollars??? Seriously???*) to print a resume that one of my roommates had designed for me. I laboriously typed twenty cover letters on a manual Smith-Corona typewriter, prayed fervently, and sent them off.

I followed up with calls to each of them – there was no such thing as voicemail, and we could not afford an answering machine in the apartment. Responses were universally discouraging, except for one. A large technology company received my letter, recorded my contact information for future reference and pitched the resume without reading it.

When I reached this one from a pay phone, I got an appointment for an initial interview. Shock and delight!

The interview went well, and most of the conversation revolved around exciting new career opportunities.

The company, in the top 50 of the Fortune 500, was growing its marketing presence rapidly and needed promising young college graduates with good communication skills to join its management development program. Although it sounded like they were looking for a golden-haired child, the pay was outstanding, and I was a perfect fit. All they needed was a drug test and my college transcript.

The drug test was no problem, but after they received the transcript and looked at my classes and grades, the conversation subtly shifted to a discussion of promising non-management positions such as building maintenance, customer service, and production line.

I should have actually read some of the Western Civ books.

From the brochure I was shown, I pointed to the customer service position because it looked like there would be air conditioning. It turned out this was the highest paying position of those offered – nowhere near the management trainee range, but regular daytime work with a credible training program and the opportunity to move up. The pay was nearly $6.00 an hour; in 1977, a real coup for a single guy with no car payment and a shared apartment.

The only hitch was that I had to pass an Assessment Center test. This was a full day of role-playing where the candidate assumed roles, first of a customer service representative and then of a sales representative. In both roles, there were interviews with company specialists playing the parts of customers, warehouse supervisors, and accountants.

Much like Captain Kirk's Kobayashi Maru exercise at Star Fleet Academy, there was no good way to win in either of those scenarios. That was the point; they wanted to see how the candidate performed in a high-stress environment. It was a wicked test and thoroughly exhausting.

As instructed, I called the employment manager from yet another noisy pay phone a week later, anticipating rejection. Instead, shockingly, she advised me that I had passed the assessment and offered me a start date.

I accepted, then immediately drove back to the dreaded bullpen office and spoke to the sales manager. I confirmed his perception that single men with college degrees were unpredictable and probably should not be hired. My tenure had lasted just over one month, and he merely rolled his eyes at my offer of two weeks' notice. I did not let the door whack me on the way out.

The new position came with three months of intensive sales training at a company facility in Dallas, all while earning this fabulous new salary plus per diem. After another three months on the job, I was promoted to management and transferred to Wichita with a 50% salary increase. Prosperity had done riz up and bit me in the rump. Best of all, I avoided the arbitrary, shallow, and poorly led management development program that had first been proposed to me. I had a real job with real responsibilities and a real risk of failure. The golden-haired children in the program had sponsors and safety nets.

A year later, I was promoted again, transferred back to Kansas City, and met my new boss, who turned out to be the devil incarnate.

Due to a management shake-up, this new boss replaced an older, long-time manager, and as often happens, felt the need to clean house. Out with the old, in with the new. Anyone associated with the previous leadership, such as a young upstart from Wichita who had been promoted twice in two years and had recently moved back to the Kansas City office, had to go.

He was overbearing, rude, disrespectful, and asinine, at least to me and a handful of others in my situation. Clearly, he wanted to make my life so miserable that I would quit. Others took the hint and began dropping like flies.

I thought, *What exactly had been so wrong with asphalt patch sales?* I was deeply offended by the injustice of this situation. I had not been with the company long, but I decided that if he thought it proper to dish it out, the best way to frustrate him was to prove I could take it.

One fateful day he called his boss to ask permission to fire me, but I knew something he did not. His boss was the one who had initially identified me as a promising candidate and was responsible for both my promotions.

Senior managers never make mistakes, and this one was not about to have one of his Chosen Few ignominiously terminated. I learned from the secretary later how the conversation had developed:

"Boss, I got a guy who needs to be gone."

"Oh? Who is that?"

"His name is Ghormley."

[Incredulous] "*Curt* Ghormley?"

And that was the end of that. Of course, the man still made me miserable, but at that point, I knew I could outlast him. So, I gritted my teeth, did my job, and helped him make his sales quota.

I could have quit, but it would have been a defeat. I was getting my professional feet under me – somewhat unsteadily – at this point in my life. I sensed that quitting would let the bully have his way. Visions of a stolen cinnamon roll in the grade school cafeteria arose, and I bristled at the reminder. I was not being persecuted for my faith; this was just business. I had not been struck backhand on the right cheek; I had been mugged in the street. They were different challenges calling for different responses.

Go away with my tail between my legs? Or hang in and take the heat? Which?

No choice. While unpleasant, I was determined not to cave. It may be unreasonable… but I'm a tough guy, you see.

Within a year, that boss was gone, promoted. On his last day in our office, I congratulated him, he scowled at me, and I smiled back pleasantly. It was a victory on par with the 11-and-1 debate tournament, except this one paid better. His parting gift to me was a punitive relocation back to Wichita. *Please, Brer Fox, don't throw me in the briar patch!* (*Uncle Remus*, Joel Chandler Harris, Peter Pauper Press, 1950.)

With a new boss and another reorganization, I was back in good graces. Unfortunately, the organization was still overly political. Many of my peers were downright obsequious in their fawning attention to senior management.

One account executive about my age, who treasured his rich mustache, heard our new vice president disapproved of facial hair. He planned to shave it off before the VP's visit later that week. When the VP showed up unexpectedly a day early (one of his favorite gotcha tactics), the account exec fled to the bathroom with a double-edge razor and shaved it off dry. *Wow.*

In that environment, there was an opportunity to move to Denver as an instructor at our National Sales School. I contemplated the move; it would be more money and considerable prestige. Or maybe not.

Our industry was in turmoil. Big players in profitable industries are always targets for competitors, regulators, and legislators. When management determines that things must change, they can sometimes change quickly. One constant every organization counts on is continued revenue from their customers... and no revenue ever comes from a national sales school. Instead, it would be a staff assignment. Most managers I knew – myself included at that point – discounted any staff work as mere marking time while the employee waited for an appointment back in the field.

Many did not want the field assignment, coming as it did with accurate metrics and the possibility of failure. This is not to minimize the value of good staff people; they make the organization run. But in my experience, there is room to hide.

I withdrew my name from consideration before an offer was made, having concluded they wanted a role model rather than an instructor. I clean up good when I wear a nice suit, but a role model, I am not.

Remaining in field business sales, I survived an endless stream of organizational changes. Finally, I found a niche in a narrow work area that most people avoided like the plague. It involved providing emergency communications services to local government agencies and was a ripe opportunity to make seriously large headlines through the failure of a very complex product. Most people were afraid of it. I probably should have been, too, but somebody had to do it.

George Patton: *Take not counsel of thy fears.*

Jesus of Nazareth: *Let not your heart be troubled.*

One day, I was in a meeting in Topeka, Kansas with a dozen other managers, including attorneys. We were dealing with new guidelines outlining legal constraints on what products and services we could offer. I had a service installation scheduled in a few weeks for a massive project we had been working on for over a year. As one small but critical part of the project, we were to provide some $50,000 of highly specialized, one-of-a-kind computer equipment. The new guidance from our corporate office was that we were not legally authorized to make that sale. It had to do with potential anti-trust litigation, and our hands were tied.

Upon receiving this news from the attorney, who was not a bad guy but often brought bad news, there was stunned silence in the conference room. This could spell doom for the project and create an enormous public relations debacle. The team leader looked around the table. "Who is going to tell the customer?" he asked quietly.

A dozen pairs of eyes turned to me, the marketing guy. I was responsible for the customer interface.

I clenched my teeth and forced a smile, gut churning. "I'll be glad to," I said. "I'll go see the customer tomorrow and let him know."

Because I'm a tough guy, you see.

At that point, I realized that if I were willing to take bad news to a high-profile customer, there would always be a place for me here.

A more significant problem loomed, however. Early in my career, it was an unexpected lesson that different people operate from different perspectives. The team leader's question, "Who's going to tell the customer?" missed the point. Being a highly adaptable corporate guy, accustomed to top-down changes in policy, he turned on a dime and accepted that the project would fail; not his fault. His question reflected his conviction that we owed the customer an honest explanation as to why we would not be able to complete his project.

So far, so good. I knew there was also the concern – maybe panic – that one of his big projects expending significant company resources for a year, would fail. It could be career-affecting.

Well, sure, it could be career-affecting, but for more than just him. Like me, too, maybe, but my perspective was entirely different. The customer, with whom I had developed a close relationship and whom I considered a mentor, had made commitments to his organization, which were now jeopardized.

What was to be *his* path forward? Trash a half-million-dollar project over $50,000 of computer parts?

Acting entirely without authority and with my heart in my throat, I contacted the equipment manufacturer directly. I got the owner to agree (through bargaining, cajoling, threatening, and pleading) to sell the equipment directly to the customer. Of course, this was way outside their business model, but he finally gave in. When I met with the customer the next day, I explained the situation. The only change was that he would issue two purchase orders instead of one: $50,000 to the computer vendor and the balance to us. The customer did not particularly like it, but he was pragmatic and accepted it.

A final detail was that I had to talk with our service manager. I explained that, although the equipment was not purchased from us, his group would be expected to maintain it. After more cajoling and pleading, he also said yes. Of course, he did not like it either, but he supported the arrangement.

This was all a little unorthodox, but nothing that compromised anyone's integrity. Call it a creative solution. Better yet, don't call it anything at all and don't talk about it. I let the team leader know the bare minimum he needed to know, and the project proceeded on track. Nobody ever asked me how these arrangements were made, and I kept my head down. It turned out there was a benefit to working in an area of the business that everyone else was afraid of.

Over the years, not every bullet was as easy to dodge as that one, but most of them worked out. Sometimes it just took a lot of creativity and persuasion to solve the problem and stay legal.

It was somewhere in there that I began to feel a vague restlessness. It was finally given voice during a morning devotional when I came across Proverbs 24:27. *Put your outdoor work in order and get your fields ready; after that, build your house.*

A house… that would mean a family, beginning with a wife. Maybe it was time.

Theological Contemplations

The Bible speaks much about the value of work. Proverbs is filled with references to work. A favorite of mine is Proverbs 6:10–11 *A little sleep, a little slumber, a little folding of the hands to rest—and poverty will come on you like a thief...*

We should not miss that many of Jesus' parables related to work. Jesus thought that work was the natural state of things. In His parables and in His outright, plain-spoken teaching, He had plenty of opportunity to commend idleness, but He did not. One reason might be that starvation was never far away, especially in that day.

A read through the Gospels finds that seemingly every other parable has a story about someone in an occupation: Farmer, fisherman, seamstress, manager, merchant, and laborer seem to be favorites. (Probably because there were not many others... no software coders or art history majors.) No doubt Jesus used these because they were expected; everybody knew approximately what each job was like and could easily relate to the story. A lifestyle of work was a widespread, common assumption.

Robert H. Bork wrote about this in his book *Slouching Towards Gomorrah.* A healthy society is characterized, Bork pointed out, by "the necessity of hard work, usually physical work, and the fear of want." *(Harper Collins, 1996, p. 8)* Sounds like something from the Proverbs.

My journey through that Fortune 500 enterprise was not about anything as big as making a healthy society. Yet, it was about more than merely paying the rent.

Chapter 3

When I experienced turmoil with my new boss, it was the first time I had ever run into serious trouble with a manager (but it would not be the last). I considered leaving the company and wondered whether it would be better elsewhere. At the time, I was strongly tempted to believe that the answer was yes, but I sensed it was not. Everybody has a boss, and in the workplace, one can find genuinely unreasonable and selfish people at any level of the organization. It was my luck to find this one only a few years into my career.

Little did I know he had a like-minded counterpart of the opposite sex whom I would have the distinct displeasure of meeting about twenty years on. *Where do they find these people?*

I think the lesson in this unpleasant encounter with the Prince of Darkness with a company I.D. was not the value of good honest work. Nor was it about the cleverness of a high school debater turned sales rep, or even the trump card of knowing the guy's boss. The value was learning that uncomfortable situations are not generally fatal. They probably can be survived, and they probably offer a model – if one has ears to hear – for surviving the next uncomfortable situation. Which will most surely come, except they never seem to get easier.

I used to pray for this man occasionally, mainly citing the passage where Jesus says, *Hard times will come in your job, but woe to the man by whom they come (My paraphrase of Luke 17:1.)* Perhaps that take on Jesus' words was not overly charitable of me.

I concluded that the actual damage a situation like this can do is to distract from one's primary occupation. The challenge to self-confidence can be debilitating; one can become so consumed with avoiding the boss (or whomever the thorn may be) that work targets are missed. Keeping the focus on the Main Event – performing the work for which one was hired – can be confusing. Yet, that is precisely what a distraction is. The proper response, I believe, requires keeping strength under control and allowing oneself to continue to be used as a channel of God's grace. It also requires self-discipline to acknowledge the challenge for what it is and meet it head-on.

Which is the definition of being a tough guy.

France, 1942

Major Paul W. Tibbets, Jr. led twelve B-17s (the Flying Fortress) in the first U.S. bombing run against German installations. The target was an aircraft factory in France in August 1942. He was flying for the Army Eighth Air Force stationed at airfields spread across the south and east of England (Three years later, Tibbets would be selected to fly the *Enola Gay,* a B-29, over Hiroshima, carrying an atomic payload to end the war with Japan.)

In September 1942, an Army Colonel, the newly appointed commander of a second bomber wing, asked to accompany Tibbets' next flight for his combat orientation. The colonel rode as an extra behind the pilot and co-pilot.

They made the bombing run without incident but were jumped by enemy fighters as they left the target area. A machine gun round burst the right-hand window from the cockpit of the Flying Fortress, put a sizable hole in the instrument panel, and set up a devastating, howling windstorm inside the aircraft.

Tibbets struggled for control of the damaged plane. Nearly deafened by the wind, he saw that the co-pilot's right hand was mangled; it was spurting arterial blood, and he would bleed out in a matter of minutes. The co-pilot held his damaged hand over his head so that Tibbets could use his own right hand to grab the man's wrist and staunch the flow. Paul Tibbets flew the plane with only one hand.

In seconds, they departed the French coast and were over the English Channel when the visiting colonel went berserk. He suddenly reached forward, pulled all four throttle levers back, and screamed that they must ditch in the Channel.

Tibbets released the co-pilot's wrist, pushed the throttles back to position, re-established control of the damaged aircraft, knocked the colonel unconscious by smashing his chin with an elbow, regained his hold on the wrist, and resumed the flight home.

In a few minutes, the visiting colonel regained consciousness, provided first aid to the co-pilot, and helped fly the aircraft. He apologized when they landed safely. (*Masters of the Air*, Donald L. Miller, Simon & Schuster, 2006, pp. 65–66.)

I often think of that scenario when I find myself in an unpleasant situation, such as when the A/C quits in the car. Or when the electric window malfunctions and will not roll up, or when I get the wrong fast-food order at the drive-thru.

*****

Psalm 118:5 *When hard pressed, I cried to the Lord; he brought me into a spacious place. (NIV)* The King James Version says, "he set me in a wide place." I asked Joel, a pastor friend – one of the most brilliant people I know – what that "wide place" meant. He speculated there was some Hebrew language behind it that was unclear. However, there were two possibilities we discussed.

One was that the lamb led to water wanted a wide field of view to see predators. The other was the warrior with a shield and broadsword who needed open space to deploy his weapon. In both cases, a wide place had a high value.

The decision to remain in a challenging situation, or escape to a different opportunity, can be stressful. Easy decision: I left the asphalt job because I would have been a fool to turn down the technology opportunity. Hard decision: On the other hand, I chose to stay with the tech outfit because I found it morally odious to leave under the terms of harassment that I faced. In time, my view of difficult managers and co-workers matured because of that experience. Apart from a few sleepless nights and mild acid reflux, I came out into a wide place. In many ways, I felt like I had survived the worst that could be thrown at me.

And that helped make me the tough guy I am today, you see.

But that experience, while a challenge, was by no means the worst.

As I would see in due time.

Chapter 4

It was 1981; I was 27, single, had purchased a modest house in Kansas City, and owned two cars and a motorcycle. The Mini Cooper was still my first love, although it was a maintenance nightmare. The more well-behaved car was a two-tone dark red ("carmine over claret," the brochure said) 1978 Pontiac Bonneville that I had bought brand new: Two-door hard top, 400 cubic inch engine, top-of-the-line accessory package.

The bike was a used Honda 750 street machine. I bought it to ride to Colorado.

The Navigators was the group that published the Topical Memory System I memorized in college. They held an annual conference retreat for people in the Wichita area who participated in their ministries. I was only peripherally involved, but I knew several people in their organization. The conference was at Glen Eyrie, their headquarters outside Colorado Springs. The main feature of the conference center was a magnificent, rambling 19th-century castle built by General William Palmer, whose statue still stands in downtown Colorado Springs.

I figured it was an excellent excuse for a vacation to the mountains on a Honda street machine.

Most of the 200-some people at the conference were married, but there were a few singles. Our meals were served family-style at 10-top tables. The first night at dinner I met Lynn, who would become my wife. She was clearly by herself.

We did not discover until later that we had a mutual friend whom I knew from high school and she from college. Stan was a little unconventional, had a motorcycle, and had taken Lynn on several junkets in the open air. When she realized I was the single guy who had come to the Nav conference on a bike (there was only one, so it was not a difficult deduction), she asked a question.

"What would it take for you to give me a ride on your motorcycle?"

I studied her. "Just a pretty smile," I said.

She offered an involuntary smile – couldn't help herself – although I suspect she and everyone else at the table rolled their eyes at the corny reply.

~~~~~~~~~~~~~~~~~~~
Other Voices

Curt and I met in 1981 at the Kansas Nav conference at Glen Eyrie. On a free afternoon, he and I went with another couple up to Eagle Lake Camp, a kids camping ministry also run by the Navigators. (Years later we sent our own boys to this camp.) It has a small mountain lake, and the setting really is quite beautiful. The staff invited us to take a canoe out. Very cool!

On the water, I mentioned "This is just like Pasquinel and McKeag!" a couple of characters from <u>Centennial</u>, by James Michener. Curt quipped right back: "Yep, a couple of crusty old fur traders from 1830." Ahh, so he had not only read the same book but liked the same characters! I wasn't thinking about dating up to this point. As far as I was concerned, Curt was just like all my other guy pals, just fun to be with. But when he said that, I thought to myself, "Hmm. This might work." – Lynn

~~~~~~~~~~~~~~~~~~~

From then on, we dated somewhat, though it required some coordination between Wichita and Kansas City. Finally, two years later, it was time to propose marriage to her. Unfortunately, I did so while we were in her rented house watching a M*A*S*H re-run. When I asked the question, she glanced my way and said, "Can we wait till the commercial to discuss this?"

But eventually, she said yes, and because I am such a hopeless romantic, I took her to a nice dinner at a unique restaurant in Newton, Kansas. There, I presented her with an engagement ring between order and salad. Fortunately, she accepted it. So on October 1, 1983, we were married in a church in Benton, a small town near Wichita, where she taught, and where we made our home. The wedding invitation said, "High noon."

We paid for the ceremony ourselves. It was a humble affair, but we maxed out that little wooden frame church building and didn't invite the fire marshall. Friends of Lynn's from Colorado (she grew up in the Denver area) brought gobs of food, and one provided photography services at cost, which was virtually nothing. The reception was in the Fellowship Hall, crowded with 30 people, and we had over 200 in attendance. Fortunately, the weather cooperated, and they spilled out onto the lawn.

What is it with this modern fixation on destination wedding venues, anyway? It is, of course, all about whether you can serve alcohol at the reception. Oh, for an earlier age when that was not an expectation. Now I sound like a fuddy-duddy. Yes, that would be me.

Lynn's brother, Ross, a warrant officer on active duty with the U.S. Army, wore his full-dress uniform. So did my oldest brother, RC, a retired Air Force Lieutenant Colonel. They happened to meet on the sidewalk before the service.

Military custom holds that when two service members in uniform meet outdoors, the junior rank initiates a salute to the senior. He is to add a greeting, such as, "Good morning, Sir," or "Good morning, Ma'am." The salute may be dispensed with if it is impractical, such as when both arms are carrying a load. Saluting indoors is not required unless one is making a report to his superior officer.

Civilians rarely get to see this except in movies, so we observed with interest the exchange of salutes, which Ross initiated. Saluting is not required if out of uniform, and probably neither one of those guys owned a decent suit. But the dress uniforms were impressive.

Because I was an up-and-coming young hotshot, I decided we would honeymoon in a far-distant state. I chose Maine partly because the wedding was in October and we could watch the leaves turn, partly because there were lots of coastlines and lighthouses in the event the foliage didn't cooperate, partly because neither of us had ever been there, and partly because they probably had outstanding New England clam chowder which we were anxious to try.

It was an expensive trip, but a completely unexpected funding source showed up. The union representing most of the workers at my company determined this was the time to go on strike. It was the end of a three-year contract, the industry was changing rapidly, and the members stopped negotiating. They walked in late August.

For us managers, it was all hands on deck to ensure continuity of service for our customers. At the time, there were only two account executives (me and the other guy) in a marketing department that had downsized by recent changes. Regarding production-related services, Mike and I were unskilled labor. We were both assigned to a company warehouse to handle hardware inventory and run orders on demand to field people working at various customer locations.

Chapter 4

We worked 16 hours a day for 20 days straight, and it was a career highlight for both of us. Of course, I would never say the time-and-a-half overtime pay, based on an already generous management salary, was why it was so much fun. Still, it would be disingenuous to claim it played no part.

On Day 20, Mike and I decided to knock off early on a Saturday night. We left work at 8:00 p.m. to get a good night's sleep. At 5:00 a.m. the following day, my phone rang. My temporary supervisor informed me that talks had settled the strike and I should not come in that day. Or any future day, for that matter. I don't think he appreciated the suits intruding into his blue-collar domain, although how he would have managed without us would be an open question.

The next paycheck had a comma in the amount and funded the entire trip to Maine. Nothing was left over, but it was an unexpected and delightful gift. The only dark undercurrent was that individuals in the bargaining unit – where I had many friends and close co-workers – missed paychecks while I was gaining one.

I should also add that the foliage was gorgeous, the lighthouse tour was intriguing – you don't get much of that in Kansas – and we got a good photo in front of one of the iconic east coast installations.

*****

Lynn and I were both 29 when we were married, established in our work and self-sufficient. There was some maturity at work which was reflected in our willingness to overlook each other's faults. That helped ease the culture shock of moving from looking out for oneself to being aware of "the other" who was suddenly living in the same house. *(Is he still here?? Why is she always here when I get home? What have I done??)*

~~~~~~~~~~~~~~~~~~~

Other Voices

I was infertile, and it made me sad; it was like carrying a heavy weight. We had faith that we could have a baby of our own, but again and again, our hopes were dashed. In my darkest moments, I questioned "Why?" All I could do was trust that God knew what He was doing. – Lynn

~~~~~~~~~~~~~~~~~~~

Given our age and the fact that we both wanted children, we were acutely aware of "The Clock" ticking away inexorably in the background. We tried but to no avail. Finally, after a year, we began inquiring about infertility.

We pursued one procedure after another but stopped short of in-vitro. The disposition of the unused fertilized eggs gave us pause. I had never thought much about this (go figure, a single guy not considering the consequences of a fertilized egg), but now I contemplated it seriously. If I believed that life was a gift of God – and I did – and that such a life was a real life from the moment of conception – and it was – then regardless of whether it happens in a petri dish or in the traditional way, we are dealing with actual human life.

As we understood it, the in-vitro process required many eggs to be fertilized to maximize the chance of success. Some are implanted, and then there are some that are frozen to be used if the implanted ones miscarried or didn't take. They are a backup plan, and their disposition becomes the question. Neither of us would have those actual human lives, even as microscopic, fertilized eggs, frozen in perpetuity or put to death. They could not defend themselves, and it seemed that killing one who was both defenseless and innocent was a sin against God and nature.

Chapter 4

God hates dishonest scales, says the Proverb. I figured that in His eyes, taking a life under such conditions would have to be balanced in some divine way, and it would come at a price I could not afford.

I called Irv, a friend who was a social worker, and asked him to find a baby for us.

He referred us to a U.S. missionary who, with his wife, was working in Guatemala. We got to know the couple and learned about their ministry. At their mission one day a few years earlier, they discovered someone had abandoned a baby on their doorstep. So, they did what anyone would do: Take the baby in, care for it, and contact the authorities and see about returning it to the mother or the mother's family, where it rightly belonged.

No such procedure existed in that country. There was no way to identify the mother or the family, so the missionary couple found themselves with a new child.

Word got around, and soon after another appeared on their doorstep. And another; and soon they were operating a full-blown informal nursery. There was no way to stop it. They made contacts in the U.S. to begin adoption proceedings.

The couple identified a new infant ready for adoption, a baby boy in their care, and put us in touch with the Guatemalan Embassy in the U.S. I contacted them. They sent me a thick bundle of required paperwork.

It was a mountain of work. It was like applying for a mortgage on steroids. They required financial statements, home studies, birth certificates (ours), proof of U.S. citizenship (ours), and so on. Everything had to be notarized, and the notary had to utilize the physical stamp to create a raised impression on the paper. Also – and I had never heard of this before – the notaries required authentication. Don't worry; there's a form. We also got fingerprinted along with the other suspects at the sheriff's office that day. *We can't be too careful where our abandoned babies are concerned!*

I spent two weeks assembling all the required paperwork, a Herculean task, double-checking everything, putting it all in a large manila envelope and sending it by certified mail to the Guatemalan Embassy. Then, finally, we were ready for our as-yet-unseen tiny Latin American, aging by the day, to join our household. Because we wanted more than one child, we had already discussed where to get a second one and agreed we would use the same path again. The kids would have physical features different from our own, but they would resemble each other, and we thought that might help them as they grew up in America.

Ten days later, I received the entire package back from the Embassy, indicating my paperwork was incomplete. I had neglected to have one of the notaries authenticated. *Sheesh!* I plowed back into the process again, obtained the proper form, requested the authentication, and received it a few days later. That night I assembled the new paperwork and decided to review it all the next day after work to make sure everything was in order, then send it off.

The next day at work, my pager buzzed; Lynn needed to talk. When I reached her, she said, "Irv called. He said a girl came into his office today, pregnant, and asked to see photos and home studies of prospective parents for her baby. Irv showed her a few and included ours, not because he thought she would be interested, but just to offer options." Lynn took a breath. "She chose us. The baby is due any day."

"I see," I said, mulling it over. "And the birth mother asked for us?"

"She did." A pause. "But the thing is, we only have two hours to let Irv know if we want it, or he will go to the next name on his list." She paused again. "Do you want this one?"

I had a couple of questions for her, which she had already posed and was ready with answers. The child was white/white (referring to the parents), there was no drug abuse, and the pregnancy had been without complication. The parents were young and unmarried, and there was at least some family stability.

I thought about the mountain of paperwork, the hours I had put in, and the unusual occurrence of overlooking a notary authentication despite my highly vaunted attention to detail. Was this a God thing? And to be fair, I also thought about the expense of a trip to Central America and the likely cash required to bring the child out.

The missionary had advised us that there would be much sitting and waiting in Guatemala, mainly for a particular passport officer to be on duty. He had done this enough times that he knew which officials were more likely to let the baby through without objection. It was a matter of "consideration" for the official. In plain speech, he advised us to bring lots of cash and be prepared to spend two weeks in-country while obtaining the child's release.

~~~~~~~~~~~~~~~~~~~~
Other Voices

After four years of frustrating treatments, we finally adopted a child in 1987, and then another in 1989. None of my big "Why?" questions were ever answered, though I had spent much time in prayer and meditation. I can't help but wonder if that experience hadn't, at least a little bit, prepared me for this ordeal with Curt and his cancer. – Lynn

~~~~~~~~~~~~~~~~~~~~

I said, "Sure, let's take the one Irv has."

Lynn was surprised, maybe shocked – *No Guatemala baby for us!* – but to her credit, she took it in stride. "Okay," she said, "I'll call him back."

We suddenly needed a baby's room and a whole lot of supplies. The thoughtful young child favored us by delaying his arrival, giving us time to get ready (*Sort of. Who is really ever ready for this?*) Two weeks later, we brought home a brand-new baby boy.

It pays to be in a small church, or maybe in a small group in a church of any size. As it turned out, we had lifelong friends there, and they wasted no time assessing and providing for our needs. A new baby in a church of 40 is a rarity, but these Christian friends outdid themselves. The women organized and held a baby shower where they deluged us with gifts: Diapers, bottles, formula, a bassinet, baby clothes, jumpers, lotions, more diapers, and all those other necessities that bewilder me.

We were suddenly parents, with a blue-lettered, "It's a boy!" sign someone had put up in our front yard.

*****

Eighteen months later, I called Irv again, looking for another child on the open market. He referred us to an attorney who was representing a mother-to-be, and we drove downtown to meet with the lawyer.

It turned out to be a less-than-happy experience where the discussion centered on money. He explained that under Kansas law, all the expenses arising out of *or during* the pregnancy were eligible for reimbursement by the adopting family.

This girl, as is common, had removed herself from her hometown for the duration of the pregnancy. She had rented an apartment in Wichita, enrolled in college classes, and needed a car.

To be crassly commercial about it (which is easy for me; *follow the money*), one can add it up: At least six months of apartment rent, university tuition, direct expenses for food and necessities, maternity clothes, and, *Oh yes*, buy her a car. Don't forget the doctor's bills; we did not ask whether she had insurance.

Chapter 4

We turned the attorney down. He was disappointed, in fact, a little rude. He told us there was a thriving underground economy for healthy white babies – call it a black market for white kids. This one could easily command $15,000 on that market, roughly twice what I had anticipated. I was not precisely offended; it just made me not want to do business with him. But I knew he was probably right.

As we left the attorney's office, we could not avoid the obvious questions: What will happen to that baby? Shouldn't we be the ones to help? What if she finds herself in a worse situation than we could provide? Isn't it worth the money to give the baby a good life?

One of the dangers of adoption is taking on a savior mentality, which we had to guard against. Letting the "I'm the only one who can help" narrative take over is too easy.

There were several false starts with other opportunities – nine in all – each unexpected, and each evaporating for one reason or another, including one particularly discouraging. In that case, we were all set to receive a newborn when, immediately after the birth, the grandmother (birth mother's mom) abruptly removed her daughter from the hospital. It was against the doctor's advice, and she refused to allow the birth mother to sign a release for the baby.

I have no idea why the grandmother did this. I suspect it was because, in her perspective, a humiliating scene was now over. The sooner everyday life returned to her family, the better. The baby, however, had been abandoned, and legal directives would now take charge. In a week, the child would enter the foster care system.

Under Kansas law, consent to adopt is invalid until the child is delivered; otherwise, it is a matter of baby selling, which is illegal. The best advice we got is that once the child is born, it is preferable to have both the mother's and father's consent. This is to avoid possible future entanglements when either party or the grandparents have a change of heart and want the child back. Sometimes this happens and can be devastating all around.

Understanding the legal issues, I was adamant that we should not present ourselves as a foster parent solution with the intent to adopt later. With no signed consent to adopt, there was nothing to keep the birth mother, her family, or the father's family (about whom we had zero information) from returning to claim the child. The threat would drag on for years. Lynn and I were disappointed but entirely in agreement with each other to forfeit this one. We never learned anything more about the situation. Savior mentality: Avoid it.

This was a gut-wrenching time. I knew little about the foster care system, but I suspected that for many children it was rife with Very Bad Things.

Make the decision, I told myself, *set your face like flint, and push on.*

Not the last time I would have an occasion to think this.

We finally got the call. A birth mother had been examined at a local emergency room after a minor car wreck and discovered she was pregnant. She was unmarried; by the time the baby was due several months later, she was in the hospital for the delivery. She declared she wished to have the child adopted. No one could locate the father, but she was willing to sign a consent form.

We learned all we could about this one after the delivery. As far as we could discern, the pregnancy had been free of complications; no drugs or alcohol were involved; the APGAR scores (a quick test performed on a baby at 1 and 5 minutes after birth) were acceptable.

The infant's pancreas had not quite started working yet, but this is not uncommon. We said yes, and our attorney obtained the birth mother's consent.

Chapter 4

Lynn spent a week near our new son while he was monitored in a special care pediatric unit while under treatment. The ailment is not serious, given adequate facilities, but it does mean lots of needle sticks and blood tests until all the internal machinery gets up to speed. Intravenous tubes and other attachments protruded from him at various places. It was heartbreaking but looked worse than it was.

Maybe the rough start toughened the kid. Twenty years later, he went U.S. Army infantry, 11-Bravo.

In a week, we brought him home to the bewilderment of his two-year-old brother who had reasonably concluded that he himself was the center of the universe. Now he was being asked to share attention with this helpless and intrusive baby. Eventually, he would be asked to carry the diaper bag. Such denigration!

Although unrelated to each other, the boys have birthdays three days less than two years apart. The older one was born on the 27th, the younger one on the 24th, and I have been confused about which is which ever since. Fortunately, I can now send both cards at approximately the correct week, which seems to work.

Imagine the difficulty explaining to a four-year-old why he is younger when it is clear that his birthday is three days *before* his brother's.

I loved being a dad. When the boys were almost two and four years old, someone asked their ages. I rounded up and said, "Two and four," and immediately suffered internal rebuke. "They are *not* two and four," I scolded myself. "They are one and three! Don't wish their lives away by accelerating their ages!" From then on, I was determined to deal with them in an age-appropriate manner, without inflation.

Grade school was a flurry of activity that accelerated as we went into middle and high school. Soccer, school projects, swimming, field trips, cross-country, academics, ADHD, Taekwondo, concerts, academic probation, homework, honor rolls, book reports, behavioral probation, broken arms, parties, required community service, cars, girls. Add to this life on the farm: We owned a modest chunk of Flint Hills pastureland that involved ATVs, shotguns, hunting, and fishing. Long-mile vacations stressed the Chevy conversion van, but the destinations were worth it: Florida beaches, Colorado skiing, Boston historicals, Gettysburg, Mount Rushmore, Texas on the Rio Grande, and others.

It's a blur, but I wouldn't trade any of it. Except maybe the shelled transmission in Pueblo. Or the broken crankshaft in Oklahoma City or the alternator in Killeen. Or, come to think of it, the melted A/C belt in Odessa, Missouri. *It's not a vacation, kids; it's an adventure!*

~~~~~~~~~~~~~~~~~~~~
Other Voices

One summer, we decided to take a road trip to San Antonio for one of Curt's conventions. The boys were around 7 and 9 years old. We packed up the van and set off one evening, taking turns driving. At midnight in Oklahoma City, the drive train broke, and a tow truck took us home. Undeterred, we set off again the next night in our trusty GMC 2-door Jimmy – a car definitely not built for long trips. Neither Curt nor I could sleep well in the small vehicle, so we found a rest stop in Texas to catch some shut eye. Curt decided to sleep on a picnic table with an old army blanket, but a few minutes later he jumped up and shook himself off, muttering about ants. They had attacked him on the table and the little critters gave him enough of a jolt to keep driving. We eventually made it to San Antonio, and it was a fun adventure we still laugh about. – Lynn

~~~~~~~~~~~~~~~~~~~~

Chapter 4

We had decided to send the kids to a private Christian school. Lynn took a job there teaching elementary and middle school band (she plays all the brass instruments, principally the trombone), which helped a little with tuition. By the time they completed private K-12, it was already like having paid for college. And then they went to college.

Before we were married, still in Kansas City, I had started working on a master's degree in Business Administration. In 1980, it was all the rage; many of my friends were doing it, and when I was single, it made sense. It gave some structure to evenings (homework) and Saturday mornings (classroom). Once married and relocated to Wichita, I had to decide whether to complete the degree. It was unnecessary for my work and would continue to take up part of my schedule.

There was little reason to finish it other than I had already put my hand to the plow. On the other hand, my employer was paying for it through a generous tuition assistance program, and before children it seemed this might be the right time to do it. So I enrolled at Wichita State University. I was, however, unprepared for what I heard from the Admissions office.

The two-plus years I already had invested (three-fourths of the required hours) were at a private university in Kansas City; the hours would not transfer. They were treated as prerequisites only, which meant I had to start over again. When I finished four years later, I had something like 45 hours in what should have been a 24-hour degree. But I got the shingle, and by the numbers, you would think I would be twice as smart.

Having spent seven years in graduate education as a student, I was surprised that when it was over, I missed it. Doing homework, reading assigned material, writing papers, and preparing for tests were much a part of my life. Six months after I graduated with the MBA, I approached Friends University about an adjunct professor position in their business school. "Adjunct" meant a part-time instructor who has a day job and only shows up on campus when class is in session. I thought of adjuncts as plastic professors.

A particular course might be offered only if an adjunct were available, and if the class attracted enough students. The university publishes the schedule, and students begin to sign up. Once the class size reaches capacity (as I recall, 24 seats), the class is declared to have "made" and is then offered to a real professor if they want to teach it. The adjunct takes the back seat.

The university offered me a Sales and Marketing class, right down my alley, and I said yes. They called me a week later. The course had made, and one of their full-time professors had taken it. Would I be interested in Money and Banking? I replied, "Sure, I've always wanted to take a Money and Banking class but never have. Sign me up."

That class was also made; another professor took it, and as a last resort they offered me Labor Problems (economics, not obstetrics; I had to ask). The class was less popular, what a surprise, and only got 20 students. Nevertheless, I took it, wondering what Labor Problems was about. I got the textbook two weeks before class and began to study. How hard could this be?

Pretty hard, as it turned out. Most of it was real Econ, which means charts, graphs, and calculus. Me, I'm a Speech major. I needed a strategy.

It would have been easy to withdraw – most of the students probably could have cared less – but I rebelled at the thought. Forward movement involves stress, I told myself. Obstacles will always and forever block the way.

So… line 'em up and knock 'em down.

Chapter 4

As a hobby, I had been reading history for several years, mainly in the form of biographies. I read about the American Revolution and then moved to the period between 1876 and 1914, post-Reconstruction to the eve of World War I. Why that? Because all the cool stuff happened then: Electricity, telephone, telegraph, big rail, big steel, big finance, stock market, Federal Reserve System, Panama Canal, Brooklyn Bridge. Henry Ford, Thomas Edison, Nikola Tesla. Grover Cleveland, the assassinations of James Garfield and William McKinley; Pinkerton, Rockefeller, Carnegie, J. P. Morgan, Teddy Roosevelt; the Spanish American War.

Building on this from books in my home library, I found excerpts related to the development of the American labor movement: The International Workers of the World (the "Wobblies"), the Haymarket Square bombing, the Ludlow Massacre, the Molly Maguires, the Pullman strike, and others. Next, I found relevant topics in the Labor Problems textbook and developed my lectures using this material. It's easy if you know the information, and everybody likes to hear stories.

I know; I'm a dweeb. I wear it proudly, but it got me through the first half of the Econ semester. This was of course nothing more than a delay tactic to get ready for the mathematics onslaught to come. I told the class that the first half would be on the history of the American labor movement, and the second half would be *(gulp)* actual economic data. Somehow, I made it through.

There is a photo of me with one of our boys, maybe two months old, sitting in my lap in a recliner at home. I have an economics textbook open, and I recall reading to him from it. I think it put him to sleep. I know it did me.

By this time, the university was on to me. For the next part-time assignment, they offered me a position as a primary instructor in an undergraduate degree completion program, which mostly avoided hard sciences like economics.

The idea was that the student in the program could finish the last two years of their bachelor's degree if they had completed at least two years of conventional education. There was a growing market for this in Wichita, as many first-line managers in the aviation industry lacked degrees. They generally had a few hours of college but sought to escape the next round of layoffs. A degree helped them avoid the Grim Reaper from HR.

The curriculum was something like 56 weeks long. A plastic professor was allowed under our accreditation to teach 48 weeks based on the modules offered. The university provided curriculum and instructor's notes, some of which I considered moderately useful under certain limited conditions. Classes were only one night each week, a four-hour session.

To break up the long classroom experience, I introduced a feature called "Slice of History." For 30 minutes each week, we discussed a historical vignette from the history of the American labor movement, shamelessly ripped from my Econ lectures. If it's your own material, it's synergism, not plagiarism. Slice of History was a highlight, at least for me. Maybe the students thought it bizarre, but at least it was entertaining and more or less on-topic.

The part-time teaching paid enough to keep up with private school tuition for the boys. I stayed with this for six years, and when the university changed the program structure, I figured my time was ending. I thoroughly enjoyed the experience, and I was able to help over one hundred students obtain bachelor's degrees (Plus, I'm a lot of fun at a party when I get started on the nuances of 19th-century American labor.) But it was time to slip away and re-focus on my primary occupation.

Concurrent with the university's change, new opportunities appeared at work. I got yet another new boss, this one a good friend of mine and a man for whom I had a great deal of respect. One of his first tasks was reviewing his new subordinates' salary structure. When he got to mine, he discovered that my compensation had moved to the bottom of the priority list because I had bounced around various organizations for several years.

Chapter 4

He corrected that in a single year and gave me a raise that fully offset the part-time income I had made at the university. Not a bad transition out of higher education.

At the same time, with new leadership at the very highest levels of our company, we became more aggressive in positioning the enterprise as a serious player in technology innovation. With my background in emergency services and willingness to remain engaged in that high-risk business, I was a natural choice to be on a winning team. Changes were coming fast.

Theological Contemplations

Proverbs 18:22 *He who finds a wife finds what is good and receives favor from the Lord.*

Commentators disagree on whether the translation should be "he who finds a wife" or "he who finds a good wife." At the Glen Eyrie castle, I stumbled across one who would be both. Good thing I had the bike along.

My grandfather found a good thing when he got married circa 1910.

Frank Ogle came to Harper County, Kansas, from Sevierville, Tennessee, in 1905 at age 15. He was the family's eldest child; at that age and in that era, it was time for him to leave the nest. Frank sold a calf for his train fare; his mother boiled a chicken and wrapped it for his trip. When he arrived in Anthony, Kansas, the chicken was gone, but he still had the same $40 cash in his pocket that he had when he left home.

Grandpa stood on the boardwalk outside the local bank, his pasteboard suitcase resting next to him, when a man approached. "Are you looking for work, son?"

"Yes, sir, I am."

"My buckboard is in front of the feed store," the man said. "Put your things in there, and I'll be along in about an hour."

And so, he was hired. He worked for this fellow for a year, and then rented an adjacent small farm from him and lived in a house on the land. He put one hundred acres to corn that year with a rented team of horses, implements, and a wagon. At harvest, he took the crop out of the field, then shelled the corn by himself, by hand.

I asked him, in wonder, "How long did that take?"

"Oh," he said, recollecting, "I started about September, and I was done 'afore the snow flew."

The following year – at age 17 – he purchased the team and wagon with the profits from the harvest, rented a second team, and did exactly the same thing again. He also made a down payment on that farm and paid off the mortgage in seven years.

Frank attended a rural church a few miles away; knowing him, he probably walked to and from to save the animals. When he was 19, there was a church social with a box dinner fundraiser.

By custom, each woman prepared a meal and placed it in a small box, concealing the contents. The men bid on the surprise dinners at auction, and the proceeds went to the church. The single girls – farm girls, every one of them – participated. They decorated their boxes to look attractive and improve the price. If a girl had her cap set for a particular boy, she would find a way to let him know which meal was hers so he could bid on it if he was interested.

Frank Ogle bought Nora McClanahan's dinner at auction for two dollars. (It was probably the most significant purchase he made that year outside of farm tools.) When he collected his meal, he approached the picnic table where she was sitting. He spoke to her. "Is this seat taken?"

She invited him to sit down; they opened the box, shared the meal, and sometime later were married. In time, she gave him a son and two daughters, the youngest, my mother.

There was a substantial monetary benefit to Frank from his marriage to Nora.

As he planted seed corn with a team of horses and a drill, Nora could walk in front, leading the team, thus straightening the rows to make them consistently close together. As a result, they probably got an immediate 25 percent improvement in yield. This, plus he no longer had to cook and clean. What's not to like?

Of course, during planting time, Nora had to prepare breakfast, spend the day in the field, mind the children, do the housework, and have dinner ready in the evening.

When Mom was still living, she told me a childhood memory of playing with her dolls under a small canvas lean-to at the edge of a field. As Dad and Mom slowly worked the horses, Nora would check on her every round.

One commentator on Proverbs 18:22 (the verse about finding the wife) has this to say in archaic KJV-speak: *Obtaineth favour of the Lord; obtaineth her not by his own wit, or art, or diligence, but by God's good providence towards him, which ordereth that and all other events as it pleaseth him.* (Benson Commentary on www.biblehub.com.)

In plain language, it means the man who finds the wife is blessed, but he does not find the wife by his own design; instead, the blessing comes from God's gift of the woman to him. It was true of Frank, and 70 years later it was true of me.

As you might surmise, I had some very dark days in the cancer ward. I cannot imagine having gone through those without my wife. There was one night when she probably literally saved my life. That was a good thing, but more on that later.

*****

Children are a gift from the Lord, saith the Scriptures (*Psalm 127:3*). Importantly, it does not elaborate on whether they are your bio kids or somebody else's. I have often thought of that Guatemalan child who was identified for us, wondering what became of him, and also the baby abandoned in the Wichita hospital at the grandmother's insistence.

Savior mentality. Don't let yourself go there, or you'll drive yourself nuts with false guilt. This very emotional and life-changing process necessitates single-mindedness. It is essential to remember that one is building a family – one family only – one is not saving the world. Single-mindedness has universal application: Finding a mate, adopting a baby, learning 16th-note rips on a tuba… or determining to fight a killer cancer from a hospital bed.

*****

"There is a tide in the affairs of men," said Brutus to Cassius in Shakespeare's *Julius Caesar,* "which, taken at the flood, leads on to fortune." His point was, literally, don't miss the boat, but it was a metaphysical reference to the appropriate time to begin a bloody revolution.

Thankfully, the bloody revolution part does not apply to my career progression. Still, at several points, I was intensely aware that I had to make decisions that would take me in new directions.

There is rarely adequate guidance for these things. No one was there to tell me whether to buy a house in Kansas City or whether to attend the Nav conference at Glen Eyrie. No one advised me whether to marry this woman or wait for another; whether to adopt this child or wait for Guatemala; whether to pursue the MBA, take a part-time teaching gig, or make any other big and small decisions. Yet, each decision we take in some way alters our future course.

The best Scripture guidance I can come up with is Isaiah 30:21. *Whether you turn to the right or to the left, your ears will hear a voice behind you, saying, "This is the way; walk in it."* This passage is Old Testament, not New Testament. In context, it cannot be taken as a hard and fast rule, but some features inform our contemporary decision-making.

"Turn to the right or to the left" implies that we move one way or the other. In the superb HBO miniseries *Band of Brothers*, there is a scene where the new recruits find themselves under small arms attack in a ditch. One of the new guys speaks to his panicked comrades, "Let's freeze!"

Just then, the seasoned sergeant jumps into the ditch and shouts, "Get moving!" They obey him and escape. Do something; don't be paralyzed by inactivity.

"Your ears will hear" implies that we remain sensitive to the Holy Spirit's leading. If one door after another seems to be closed, the right answer might be to retreat and go the other way. Recall the Apostle Paul's journey through Asia Minor, which we would call Turkey, toward the west and the Aegean Sea (*Acts 16*). The Spirit continued to push him westward until he came to the sea's edge and could go no further. That was when "the Macedonian man" appeared to him in a dream and called him to come across the water to Greece.

I am not recommending that we wait for a dream to give guidance, but once having moved, it is vital to listen for the Spirit's leading.

Don't miss this part: His leading may come in many ways, including closed doors, opened doors, or counsel from a mature Christian.

"This is the way, walk in it" suggests that once we have determined the correct course, we stay with it and make it work. That does not mean the path will be easy; it may be incredibly challenging. A rugged jeep trail on a four-wheeler will show clearly that a hard trail is not the same as a closed trail. In life's challenges, Christian maturity demands knowing the difference.

In a hospital bed with complications arising from leukemia, there were multiple occasions where the experience was so hard – the pain so intense – that the temptation to let go was strong. But I did not, and I also did not spend much time in those moments contemplating Isaiah Chapter 30. I had already contemplated Isaiah 30, thank you very much, and had determined that if there were any way to do so, I would exert every possible effort to survive.

Because I'm a tough guy, you see.

It did not keep me from longing for the rest and lasting relief that the next act would surely bring; but that was God's deal, not mine.

Belgrade, Yugoslavia, 1939

Love stories and courtships have often accelerated during wartime, particularly in Europe, where the Nazi menace spread rapidly in the 1930s and '40s. Gregory A. Freeman documented one marvelous story in *The Forgotten 500* (NAL Caliber, 2007). He offers a remarkable account of the rescue of U.S. bomber crews of the 15th Air Force operating from various airfields in the Mediterranean area who were shot down over Yugoslavia.

It is a love story begging for a network streaming series.

American-born George Vujnovich, of Serbian heritage, studied medicine in Belgrade in 1935 where he met Mirjana, a local student. Immediately taken with her poise, intelligence, and beauty, George tried to strike up a relationship with her.

George's brash American style was too abrupt for the Serbian girl, and she brushed him off. In a few months, she received a scholarship to study abroad at Cambridge, an envied opportunity, and left for England. George, heartbroken, concluded he would never see her again.

Chapter 4

When Mirjana returned to Belgrade in 1939, they met again, at a party, renewed their acquaintance, and began dating. George learned from his earlier mistake and proceeded more cautiously. The young couple fell in love with rumors of war abounding. For a time, Belgrade was left unscathed, but then, disaster. Because of Yugoslav reluctance to fully cooperate with the Third Reich, Hitler ordered the city bombed in early 1940. With their city in ruins and homes demolished, the civilian population predictably panicked, and thousands fled the country.

Mirjana had no passport and would not be allowed to leave. Worse, she had been identified as a potential spy because of her time at Cambridge, and thereby came up on Nazi lists.

George found a willing priest and a friendly government official; George and Mirjana were married secretly, the marriage license issued, and they could now travel under George's American citizenship.

Following a circuitous and harrowing route, Mirjana escaped to America where she found employment as a translator in the Yugoslavian Embassy in Washington, D.C. By this time, the U.S. was in the war. The OSS, forerunner to the CIA, recruited George and stationed him in Italy. As with many couples during wars, these two were apart for the duration of hostilities.

One day, a memo came across Mirjana's desk. A source had identified some 100 downed U.S. airmen hiding in a village in Yugoslavia who were being protected by local resistance fighters. Outside of official channels, she sent word to her husband. George notified his superiors, who tasked him to organize a rescue effort.

What followed was nothing short of miraculous.

George Vujnovich recruited a three-man team of U.S. operatives of Serbian descent to parachute into the mountainous area near the village. They engaged the flyers – now 250-strong – and local residents to convert a mountain pasture into a 700-yard-long airstrip for C-47 transport planes. They had virtually nothing in the way of tools; they used bare hands and ox carts to dig out rocks and fill in the dirt. The aviators all understood what a runway needed to look like and took care to make it as smooth and solid as possible. By the time it was ready (an optimistic assessment), there were over 500 airmen whom the resistance had routed to their location.

During this time, a German Wehrmacht battalion, with perhaps a thousand hardened Nazi troops, was ensconced less than five miles away.

Carrying a dozen men at a time, C-47s flew in and out of the tiny airstrip over the course of one night, wheels brushing dark treetops on the way out. The Germans never detected them, no casualties occurred, and no aircraft were lost. Outrageously daring, it was, and is still, the largest military rescue in U.S. history.

The marriage of George and Mirjana, arranged so hastily and under such unlikely conditions, lasted 62 years until the death of Mirjana in 2003.

Having made a commitment to one another, George and Mirjana never abandoned it, and hundreds of others, and their families, were benefactors.

He who finds a wife finds what is good and receives favor from the Lord.

Chapter 5

My career swerved into its first big detour in 1998, and I learned a profound life lesson the hard way, a lesson that would pay big dividends even as it cost me money. *In their hearts humans plan their course, but the Lord establishes their steps (Proverbs 16:9).*

Confession time: I do get mightily tired of learning lessons. Surely, I could just watch a YouTube video to learn serious lessons, but that doesn't seem to be the way it works. In any event, after this development was fully cooked in my mind, it yielded guidance that was useful even in battling leukemia. And frankly, anything useful in battling leukemia – or any other disaster of life – is worth considering.

For 15 years of my early career, I had been selling and implementing emergency communications systems for municipalities across Kansas. Most of the customers got to know me and trusted me; our products and services were priced reasonably, and while the compensation plan was mostly salary rather than commission, it paid well, and I had no complaints.

I was successful, and the company I represented was successful. I ended up with about fifteen subordinates through minor organizational tweaks, and we made a good team. I was a second-line manager, meaning I had first-line supervisors reporting to me, with non-management personnel reporting to them.

The future was nothing but bright until the next reorganization. Storm clouds gathered. In this restructure, management ignored the specific needs of the emergency communications market segment and instead arranged head count based on the scope of the larger organization.

Who would ever think an organization chart should reflect the needs of the actual business segment involved? This was probably the brainstorm of one of those golden-haired children in the management development program.

Where there were three second-line managers in Kansas (myself in Wichita, Frank in Topeka, and Leon in Kansas City), the new org chart called for only two. The locations were unimportant as the work could be managed from any of those offices. At the same time, a new second-line position was created in Wichita in an entirely different section of the company. Because of the large number of people reporting to it, that job had to be done in Wichita.

One of us in the emergency sector would have to go.

I was senior, had upper management support, and considered myself safe. But the new position had to be staffed in Wichita. If I insisted on remaining in my present work and location, the new job would be filled with a promotion from another quarter. No problem there, but either Frank or Leon, both of whom I liked and had worked with for years, would be forced into early retirement.

Knowing those guys, I could have found my tires slashed *(Just kidding. I think.)*

At this point, it would have been most helpful if someone had told me that just because there is a high road doesn't always mean it's necessarily the right road. Nevertheless, I accepted the job transition, took the new Wichita position, and left the emergency communications sector behind. My buddies were safe and remained employed.

*****

Chapter 5

I met with my new organization – 121 unimpressed faces in eight work groups – and spent the next month learning what they did. I was stuck in an office; no more road trips for me and no more worshipful customers glad to see me or ready to take a chunk out of my hide (I relished both).

In the new business, any customer escalated to me had such a complaint that neither the telephone rep nor the first-line supervisor could solve the problem.

Oh, joy.

My new boss was in Texas, the center of the universe, just in case there was any question about that. She appeared to be disdainful of us who dwelt in the hinterlands; and from the beginning, she and I did not have a warm relationship. I think I was the wrong age, color, and sex (maybe all three), but that's only a guess. It may have been because she was intimidated and insecure. *Me? Intimidating? Surely not.* But I am not inside her head and was not then, and she probably had good reasons for acting the way she did.

We who reported to her had frequent group conference calls with her on *her* schedule, which was frequently at 5:00 p.m. They lasted for an hour or two and were generally not scheduled until earlier the same day. The boss apparently did not have to get home for dinner.

Six months after joining this new group, there was yet another organizational shift in the emergency communications sector, which I observed only from a distance. They needed a new third-line manager because the company had decided to build the enterprise into a high-profile part of the business. I would have been in a perfect position to take that promotion and may have been asked… but I was no longer on their org chart.

Oh well.

Twelve months after joining this new group, my buddies, whose jobs I had protected at such significant personal cost, left the business. Frank retired, and Leon found a sweet position as a spokesman for a not-for-profit group in Kansas City. *Oh well. Again.*

What doesn't kill you will make you stronger.

About that time, we got a new Vice President – *New ideas, Oh, goody!* – and in an unexpected move, I learned that my high activity customer service representatives would be terminated en masse. They handled the most high-profile customers in our segment, and their work was to be farmed out to a colossal, and, in my humble opinion, incapable service rep population in Dallas.

I had 25 people in that group in Wichita; the Dallas crowd was over 200. Staff had determined that the business could be run more efficiently by consolidating the groups and that the enormous Dallas office could pick up the work without additional headcount or effort. This was of course not true, but the only people who would notice would be my 25 reps put out in the cold, and our influential, loyal customers spread across Kansas.

Who cares what the customers think? The golden-haired children have spoken.

I contemplated calling my boss but sensed it would do no good. So I called the staff guru instead. He was a solid thought-leader who had had no role in this proposed shift. "Jim," I said, "you know this is wrong. My Wichita people have an average of 20 years with this company and provide top-of-the-line service to these customers. They are the highest-trained, most competent people of their title in this state. Where do you expect them to go?"

"Can't solve that problem," he replied. "You know this wasn't my idea. I know you're probably disappointed, but the decision has been made." He paused. "The work will transition on November 15th. You will be required to notify them, per union rules, on that day and not before."

Chapter 5

"'Disappointed' does not do it justice, Jim. You're going to make me surplus those people ten days before Thanksgiving?" I asked incredulously. "This company does not do things like that. But here's another thing," I said. "In Wichita, these people have no career path upward. We are such a small organization that once a service rep gets into this group, they cannot reasonably expect another promotion. That's why they have 20 years of service with us. The last time anyone in that group submitted a transfer request was years ago.

"Think about this," I pressed. "All other company positions are available to that group in your Dallas office." I swallowed and played my trump card, hoping it would be enough. "I talked to the unit manager in Dallas. He tells me the morale is so low that the average length of tenure in that group is 18 months. And you know what that figure represents."

There was a pause. "I do."

"I know you do. Per union rules, a service rep must remain in the title for a minimum of one-and-a-half years before submitting a request for transfer. Jim, everyone who joins that group wants to get out as soon as possible. There is no longevity; there are no old hands; there is no one with anywhere near the experience level to handle these customers effectively." Again, I paused and threw out the request: "Jim, I would ask you to talk to the VP and get this decision overturned."

There was a long silence, and then, "Curt, it can't be done. The decision has been made and will not be changed." This, more than anything, convinced me he had already made these or similar arguments and lost the battle. He softened his voice. "I am truly sorry for your people and the position you are in. I know you didn't ask for this, and neither did they, but this is how it will have to be."

And that was that.

Until the next day. *We do not always get to choose the trials we face; only how we face them.*

I continued working the phone, calling in favors and snooping for information. I called Jim again, and he was not happy to hear my voice. "What is it now, Curt? You know I can't change that decision."

"Something entirely different, Jim," I responded. "You know the plan you guys have to move that Billing Inquiry Unit out of Houston?"

"Yes," he said cautiously. "We've discussed it. Why?"

"I've talked to the unit manager there. She has 35 people in her group, which is being disbanded and absorbed into another area. She needs to transition the billing work to someone else."

"You're not telling me…" he began.

"I want it here," I said. "I have 25 trained, experienced service reps who will be available for the assignment in January. They come with two supervisors. I will take the Billing Unit into my group and manage it for you; you will have to transfer ten new headcount to me to complement the people."

There was a pause. "We weren't going to move on that 'til the first quarter."

"Jim, January *is* the first quarter. I will set up a conference bridge with the Houston group, and you and I can propose the plan and develop a timeline."

"We'll have to get it approved."

"I have every confidence in you, Jim. Do some of that special staff magic and make it happen. Please."

I let my first-line managers in on the plan and swore them to secrecy. They did not exactly take it in stride. "What!!??" one of them shouted. "You want to destroy one of the most effective groups in this company and turn them into a Billing Complaint Desk??"

"A Billing Inquiry Center," I corrected, "and please try to remain calm. Remember your condition." Her face was red, and she did not take the humor as well as I had hoped. "There are no other options," I said. "I'll give you time to process this but know that we are probably headed for this change. Your people won't like it – heck, I don't like it either – but we will not be able to change it. The best we can hope for is to protect their jobs and avoid a surplus condition."

They eventually calmed down, and after extracting further assurances of their silence, I turned them loose. I could have used a shot of bourbon right then, but it was just my luck that I didn't drink.

A week later, I spoke with Jim again. "I am waiting for your official announcement," I said. "I have to announce this to the group tomorrow. I want to tell them about the Billing Center at the same time I tell them they are losing the high-activity accounts."

"We are still waiting on the Vice President's approval," he said, "but the timeline has been extended. You are now to wait another ten days to make the announcement. Hopefully, you can do both at the same time."

"Jim," I said, "that's almost Thanksgiving! You're cutting that a little close, aren't you?"

"That's better than the alternative," he said. "At least we are still in the game." He paused. "Are you sure you want the Billing Inquiry Center in your shop? It's a tough job."

"Jim, I don't want to be anywhere close to it. But somebody's got to do it, and we can make it work."

"Will you get pushback from your service reps?"

"Count on it. But Jim," I added, "they are good people and will step up when I ask them to do it." And I meant it. I had always been truthful with them, sharing what information I could. While demanding high performance, I had always attempted to be fair.

"Okay, I'll see what I can do."

"Jim, I'm afraid you'll have to do a little better than that. Next week, I am going to tell them both sides of this transition: They are leaving the high activity group and moving to the billing group."

"I told you; it's not approved yet." He was beginning to sweat. I thought, *Good.*

"Make it happen, Jim. We are going to do this."

A week later, I called a meeting with the high activity reps, all hands, for 8:30 a.m. on the Wednesday before Thanksgiving. Just in time, I received an email from my boss approving the organizational change I had insisted on. However, she never commented on why the change was being made; I got the impression she was washing her hands of it.

I met with the service reps as ordered and gave them the news. "First," I said, "your high activity account responsibilities are being transferred to our Dallas office. We will transition beginning next week." There was a stunned silence before the groans and complaints began.

I held up my hand. "You will be allowed to call your customers and explain the situation. The phone system will be redirected so that all their calls will automatically go to Dallas by mid-December. I know you don't like this but understand that I will expect – demand – a high degree of professionalism from each of you." I surveyed the sober faces. "And I will personally be observing your calls, listening in on you randomly. Do not disappoint me in this."

One raised their hand. "Yes?"

"If our work goes away, what happens to us?" There were murmurs; this was the elephant in the room.

"Well," I said, "I have good news and I have bad news. The good news is you are the new Billing Inquiry Center for the Texas market, and you all still have jobs with your same title, and your same rate of pay." More groans. They understood this better than I did. "The bad news," I glanced around the room, "is that you all still must work for me. I will continue to be your unit manager."

"Do you know anything at all about billing?" the questioner asked, scoffing. There were sniggers.

"Not a thing," I admitted. "But I'll bet we both do in a month."

Predictably, zero appreciation came my way from the group for my machinations. They never knew how close they had come to losing paychecks. I left it that way and never brought it up.

*****

Handling billing inquiries was indeed the Complaint Center. Calls sometimes got very heated as customers who could not pay their bills were in contact with my reps. It was an entirely different environment for our people and sometimes quite unpleasant. But the work had to be done, and the customers had to pay the bill one way or the other. Eventually, we learned to take it in stride.

There was one development, however, about which I had serious ethical issues. Our new Vice President, to whom my boss reported, suddenly ordered that we discontinue refunds to customers. I learned his compensation was partly based on reported net revenue, so any substantial refund worked against his paycheck.

Some of these large accounts had billing errors above $50,000. It did not cost our company money; these were nothing more than bookkeeping discrepancies, as we were the billing agent for third parties.

Most of the third parties were new to the industry, attempting to take advantage of new regulatory freedoms to carve out what they hoped would be a profitable market niche. Some of them made honest mistakes, while I was convinced that others were outright fraudulent. Nevertheless, a refund for that amount exceeded my level of authority, but not that of my boss. When I got one of these, I would routinely submit it to her attached to an email and obtain her authorization to refund.

With her new direction from the Vice President, her refund authorizations came to an abrupt halt.

I'm sorry... what was that?

We owed the billing correction to the customer and simply refused to make it. To be clear, there was no money involved (other than the VP's compensation check); for us it was mere recordkeeping, but for the customer it was real accounts payable. If they ignored it, it would be turned over to a collection agency.

After the first refund was ignored – incredibly – I began keeping meticulous documentation, on hard copy, in a safe place, not on company property. The worst was one for $86,000 for a large customer enterprise in Texas. It was a legitimate request, and my emails and phone messages to my boss were met with silence. She ignored the issue. I began to grind my teeth.

Look, lady, I thought, *the reality is what it is. Let's face up to it!*

(Does that sound like cancer? Actually, yeah, maybe so. But at the time, it was the furthest thing from my mind.)

This had lawsuit written all over it. Within a week, I called a senior manager in the emergency communications organization and asked if he had a job opening. The answer was yes, and a month later I found myself back over there, although in a different capacity from when I had left.

I was, of course, still an employee, and soon after that move, I got a call from a company attorney. Unsurprisingly, there was legal action pending. He asked if I knew of an $86,000 refund request that had come out of my group. As a matter of fact, I did. I retrieved the paperwork and sent it to him.

A few days later, my former boss was off the payroll.

Too bad for her; but think about it – with her departure, her customers were better off, her managers were better off, and I was better off. The new person promoted into her position was better off; she retired and was better off. Besides that, the people she served in the new small business she launched were better off.

I should have asked that "Who will be better off?" question before I accepted the move out of the emergency group in the first place. Don't misunderstand me; I didn't lose my paycheck and I still had a career, so all was good. But the detour I had taken was an unnecessary interruption.

*****

Once back in the emergency communications end of the business, things straightened out for me. My initial assignment was a simple job coordinating our product implementations. At the first opportunity, I called my new boss, who was in a different state and had never heard of me. I introduced myself.

"I know you didn't pick me for this job," I said. "I know you were handed me because I called our Vice President directly and asked for a position." He grunted with acknowledgment.

"I want you to know that I will not be a problem child." I went on, "I plan to do this job, keep my head down, and not cause you any grief. You didn't get to choose your own guy – which you probably wanted to do – but I'll try to ease your pain by making myself a non-issue."

He was surprised, but I think gratified by the call. I had been in situations like this myself where I had been "gifted" with an employee from upper management. In a large organization, these appointments are often a dumping ground for a problem. While I knew my new boss would be suspicious of me, I did not need his help with the work; mostly, I wanted him to look elsewhere for problems to solve.

He and I became good friends, and in later assignments, we worked closely together. Sparks occasionally flew, but this beginning laid a good foundation for trust.

My new gig eventually became the old gig on steroids. In two years, I was appointed sales manager in the emergency communications arena handling some very substantial municipalities. (Some of these were snake pits of local politics, but one takes the good with the bad.) Unfortunately, as was perennially the case, we were understaffed for the job before us. I had only eight subordinates, all highly proficient technical salespeople; but the sudden expansion of new technologies and IP (Internet Protocol) features was overwhelming. There were also new competitors we had not seen before in our field.

The great thing about a free market is that somebody always comes up with a fresh way to disrupt your business model. *With my skills and your customers, I could take your customers away from you.*

My people were so engaged in designing, selling, and implementing complex systems – exactly where they needed to be – that some of the more tedious activities had the potential to fall by the wayside. It was up to me to see that they didn't. Most of my time, therefore, was spent on contract negotiation, supplier relations, inter-departmental conflicts, resource allocation, and weekly, monthly, and quarterly reports to management.

Much of the job involved problems that had no good solutions, and nearly all required making decisions with incomplete data. Risks had to be balanced against penalties and rewards, and quickly: Multiple actors – competitors, over-zealous regulators, and vendors with sudden new technologies – allowed no leisurely reflection to determine strategy.

I did not suspect it at the time, but responding to a sudden ambush by an unseen cancer would be uncannily similar. Except the stakes were higher.

And trade shows: Every state had an annual trade show where suppliers were expected to show up (and pay for the show), and all our customers were in attendance. In addition, there were a couple of national trade shows where we were a key supplier, displaying a presence with an elaborate booth in the vendor hall.

At a certain point, my counterpart sales manager in California retired early and unexpectedly. His organization matched my own in terms of employees and customer base. His departure occurred a few days after the internal security team opened an investigation into improper gifts to company employees from vendors. That was perhaps just a coincidence, or maybe he got caught up in something out of his control. I can say I didn't know anyone with more integrity, but he was suddenly gone.

I contemplated what this change would mean to our organization, and then approached my boss: "I know what you're about to do," I predicted. "You have a vacancy in California that you are about to fill by promoting one of my people, probably from the Texas market."

"I have thought about it," he admitted. "You have some very good people."

"Yes," I agreed, "and none wants to be a sales manager or move to the Left Coast. But you will convince somebody to take one for the team – just as you did me when I took this thankless job – and then, because of budget constraints, you will not backfill him in my team."

He smiled. "There are always budget constraints."

"So, I will have to rearrange my already thin group, disrupting relationships with some of our flagship customers. Then you will ask me to mentor the new guy in California – he is my guy, after all – so that he can compete against me for sales results."

"That sounds like a good plan," he replied, still smiling.

"So, if that's the case," I countered, "why don't you just give me the California territory in addition to what I already have? It will double my quota, but it will also double the opportunities, and it will allow you to redeploy the headcount somewhere else."

And that's how it went down. The headcount was indeed deployed somewhere else – not in my area. I began traveling to California in addition to Texas; I flew every week and in no time became a million-mile flyer on American Airlines. There was essentially no impact on my income, but because of the time zone difference, the length of my work days went from 10 hours to 12.

On one particular trip to Los Angeles for a trade show, I rode an airport shuttle bus with only one other passenger, our customer. He discovered I was the new sales manager and said, "Oh, good, glad to meet you! I'll come by the booth later and bust your chops!"

"I look forward to it," I said. "It's always good to be back in California!"

"Yeah," he replied dryly as he watched the scenery go by. "Welcome to the People's Republic of…"

*****

With everything else going on, one incident was truly frustrating because it was a complete distraction and could not be ignored. In one of the geographic areas we served, a high-ranking state law enforcement officer contacted my office asking my input on methods for prioritizing new technology upgrades in his department. For a sales manager, this is like being invited into the candy store with a free gift card.

Chapter 5

When I arrived at his office – involving an out-of-town trip and yet more overnight travel – I found myself meeting with the official plus three aggressive competitors, all in the same room, all of whom were angling for my dominant market share. It turned out that the officer was working on his MBA and needed to write a lengthy essay on – you guessed it – methods for prioritizing new technology upgrades in his department. He sought input from each of us.

I was expecting a half-day discussion of current technology systems, departmental goals, identified problems, and potential solutions. In fact, the meeting lasted less than thirty minutes. He made the assignment, provided his assistant's email address, and asked us to submit written recommendations within a week based on our extensive and invaluable experience.

Clearly, the assistant would be tasked with synthesizing the responses into a seamless document – without attribution – suitable for submission to his professor. This, like the meeting itself, would no doubt be on company time using state resources. It would be an understatement to say this was an unthinkable violation of ethics.

We looked at each other, deadpan, and left the premises separately to go write his homework for him.

I contemplated pushing him down the stairs. But only briefly.

Line 'em up and knock 'em down. It's not like I hadn't cranked out term papers before.

While it was an enormous distraction, had absolutely nothing to do with sales and would not contribute a dime to my quota, this request – coming as it did from a decision-maker with contractual authority – could not be ignored. I later considered how much it resembled leukemia: The cancer by itself will not kill you, but the unscrupulous actors it lets into your system, if left unaddressed, most certainly will.

*****

That sales manager assignment was a hectic, wild ride – every supplier with a self-proclaimed fantastic IP-based product proposal assaulted California and Texas. My time was spent helping the two teams meet that competitive pressure. We, too, had an extensive suite of IP products, of course, but the challenge was overcoming inertia. Some of our people were accustomed to comfortable repeat business and were surprised when they lost an account.

One of my sales reps complained, "Our vendors, who are supposed to be supporting us, are going around us to the customers. They're announcing new products without talking to us first. I want you to tell the vendors to stop that!"

So now I'm supposed to tell somebody else's sales organization *not* to see a customer? (Several potential responses come to mind, all quite crass.) "Here's an idea," I told him, a little short on patience, "why don't you get out to your customers first and let them know that *you* can bring the products to them?"

My guy had a right to be frustrated, but the problem he had identified was not new, was not unique to our industry, and could not be solved. The only way to fix it was to be more aggressive than the vendor. We had to show our supplier that his best opportunity was to sell his products through our already-established relationship. Be bold, strong, and competent; the vendor will probably fall in line. Meekness, not weakness!

*****

Chapter 5

I managed these two territories for five years and then decided to let someone three decades younger take over. I announced my retirement to my boss privately one year before my departure. Six months later, I announced the departure internally and to customers with whom I had worked closely.

I worked at the same pace – fast, focused, effective – until the last day. Near the end of a career, many people I knew joined the RIP program, "Retired in Place." I frankly resented it and was determined to show a different way.

On September 30, 2013, I left my office for the last time. On October 1, 2013, I started delivering firewood.

*****

I had purchased a small firewood operation from Gene, a local guy a few years older who was ready to get out. He sold high-quality products to high-end residential customers, and I liked his business model.

Wintertime sales were traditional firewood, delivered by pickup with a wheelbarrow and lovingly stacked by hand for the customer. Summertime sales were smoking and grilling woods sold wholesale to area merchants. Gene built the business with high integrity and demonstrated maximum effort for each customer. No day was too cold nor nasty to deliver firewood, and no smoking woods order was too big nor demanding.

That focus was admirable, and I continued in the same vein. I also worked my soft American Airlines tail off and dropped 30 pounds in the first two months. I had it to lose. One morning in January, having just loaded the pickup in a winter blizzard, I called Gene, raising my voice into the phone to be heard over the diesel engine and the raging wind. "I do not recall 11 degrees Fahrenheit and sideways snow being in our contract!"

"Check the fine print," he responded, yawning, while watching the storm outside his patio door. "Have your people call my people, and we'll work it out."

The nice thing about semi-retirement was the freedom in the schedule. I joined Lynn in the community band she had played in for years, and also picked up other (mostly unpaid) gigs and small ensembles as time permitted: Dixieland jazz, brass choir, brass quintet, some on-demand holiday concerts. It was good to be on the input side of a tuba again, but I had to hustle to keep up. Fifty years of neglect requires some focused attention to overcome. Tubby wanted his revenge.

Lynn and I planned a trip to Europe for the following year where we would spend almost two weeks in England and France. I blew my entire stash of American Airlines and Hilton Honors points on airfare, hotel, and a rental car. They were all free.

Which meant it was only a multi-thousand-dollar trip out of pocket. I'd still like to know who gets the $400 tax per ticket for flying over the ocean. Actual payment required, not travel points.

~~~~~~~~~~~~~~~~~~~~

Other Voices

Curt and I were both fortunate to have attended high schools with excellent music programs. He played tuba and I played trombone and euphonium.

Professional-level instruments are expensive, and tubas especially. I purchased my "good" trombone when I was in college and still play the same horn today. Curt never had his own tuba; schools typically provide those expensive instruments for students. After college, whenever he had a chance to play, he was always saddled with some old clunker that looked like it had been assembled from spare parts in the junk room.

A lot of guys, when they retire, buy a boat or a car. Not Curt! He bought a brand-new professional-line tuba! And yes, there is a monetary equivalent with a boat or car.

With the new tuba, he began playing in the community band. It was fun to play in the same group together. He was so into it he offered his truck and trailer to help move equipment to and from our performances. During the 2022 concert season, I began to think he was sure aging faster than I was. He looked worn out and lacked energy. He was 68, after all, and old age catches up with all of us. At an outdoor performance (Naftzger Park, downtown Wichita), he drove the truck but told the director he was too tired to help move equipment. That was June 21.

His annual wellness exam was scheduled for the next morning.
– Lynn

~~~~~~~~~~~~~~~~~~~~~

We spent the first week in London, traveling by tube and on foot, and saw as many of the touristy sites as we could: Buckingham Palace, Windsor Castle, Hyde Park, Churchill's underground war room, Westminster Abbey, Piccadilly Circus, Paddington Station (but there was no bear in sight), crown jewels at the Tower of London. We climbed the 528 steps to the top of St Paul's Cathedral.

Windsor Castle is accessed by first entering the Guard's Room, where an enormous artistic wall display confronts the visitor. It is composed entirely of retired flintlock pistols, hundreds of them, meticulously arranged in a beautiful mosaic. The message is clear: We have arms to spare; don't mess with us!

After a week in London, we took the overnight ferry from Portsmouth to Caen, a six-hour transit across the Channel. Despite my highly touted management experience, I chose not to pre-plan the Normandy excursion. I figured that if I made all the arrangements earlier, we would regret having missed locally available opportunities. Unfortunately, these did not present themselves, so I worked the hotel phone one day for three precious vacation hours looking for English-speaking lodging in France.

I found a place near Sainte-Mere-Eglise, which, thanks to The History Channel, was the only place name I recognized in Normandy. At the cathedral there, U.S. paratrooper John Steele's parachute snagged on the church spire as he descended early on D-Day morning. Steele remained suspended in effigy 70 years later as a tribute to the U.S. 505th Parachute Infantry Regiment. In 1944, the unfortunate Steele hung in his harness for hours as the battle raged beneath him. I remember him best as Red Buttons in *The Longest Day* (1962).

With everything finally arranged for the France trip, we spent the last day in London sightseeing.

Thanks to the Hilton Honors account, we could keep our hotel room in Ealing (on the west side of the city but near a tube station) while taking the side trip to France. This would allow us to leave most of our luggage and bring only day packs.

I told Lynn we needed to leave the hotel at 7:00 p.m. to catch the tube, the train, and the ferry. At 5:00 p.m., we returned, exhausted from the day, ready to shower and pack... and I thought about it.

"Dear," I said, "I was slightly wrong about the schedule. The train *leaves* at 7:00 p.m., and we must get to the station first, and this is rush hour. This means," I swallowed, "we need to leave here in fifteen minutes."

A flurry of packing, a call for a black cab, mounting dread. To my wife's credit, she took it in stride. *It's not a vacation; it's an adventure!*

Chapter 5

With us aboard, the taxi crowded onto the main street, which resembled a parking lot. We crawled at a snail's pace. At the train station, we were unsurprised to find we would miss our schedule. At length, we finally discovered a human ticket agent – not a machine – who could show us a different route. We hopped a train to a town I had never heard of, changed to another train, and arrived at the ferry – hungry, frazzled and a little panicked – at 11:00 p.m., a bare ten minutes before departure.

See there? Can I manage a schedule, or what?

Relieved to have made the ferry, I left Lynn to doze and found my way to the restaurant, which had closed for the night at 10:00 p.m. *(On an overnight ferry??)* The casino was, of course, open 24 hours, so I took a seat at the bar and asked what sandwiches they had.

"We don't serve food after 10:00 p.m. Only drinks." Of course. It was probably the same kitchen that served the restaurant.

"No peanuts? Pretzels?"

"No, nothing. Just drinks." The bartender shrugged and turned away to serve more promising customers at the other end of the bar.

I found a vending machine and purchased a suspicious ham sandwich and a bottle of water. There was no mayonnaise. *It's not a vacation; it's an adventure. Remember Paul Tibbets in his B-17.*

*****

France: Finally, a country where they drive on the *right* side of the road! I had been unwilling to trust my instincts in England, so we traveled by tube and taxi while there. Impractical in rural France, I was glad to rent an Avis car. I was even more glad I could operate a standard shift transmission, as choices seemed limited.

After a sleepless night on the ferry, we circumnavigated the city of Caen on the highway loop three times studying inscrutable exit signs in French. At length, we chose one that seemed to promise westward. We eventually found our way to our bed and breakfast, a quaint four-story firetrap with a tiny parking lot for tiny cars and a garden wall 600 years old. Really. It was one of the few structures in town that had survived D-Day.

As we drove through the Normandy countryside in the following days, it seemed that every farm home had a museum attached. The owner had found a dented helmet and perhaps a mildewed canteen cover or a few discarded M1 Garand stripper clips in his field and monetized them with signs in English claiming, "Invasion relics! WW2 history! We love Americans!" One small town on the coast boasted a visitor's center with similar "We love America!" sentiments posted... but no one on their staff had a word of English. *An odd way to show it*, I thought.

The invasion beaches interested us, but the American Cemetery at Colleville-sur-Mer was the most remarkable... an incredibly humbling experience.

We spent three days in the country, then took the ferry back to England, the train to London, a couple more days of sightseeing, and flew home. It was a trip worth remembering. I still have visions of 9,386 white crosses lined up in perfect military symmetry overlooking Omaha Beach, mute testimony to the cost of freedom.

*****

Eventually, I concluded that while entertaining and healthy, the firewood business was not especially lucrative. So, I went back to work for a small company in Wichita – one of my wholesale firewood customers – selling meat processing equipment and supplies to butcher shops and slaughterhouses. My territory was Pennsylvania and New England. I traveled one week a month and thoroughly enjoyed it.

When I was interviewed for the job, one of the questions was, "Seeing you have already been a sales manager for a huge company, how will you like being merely a sales rep in a small business?"

"I think it will be like a paid vacation," I said, and I meant it. And it was.

*****

The other significant development during this time involved our church. Early on, Lynn and I decided that our kids would attend a private Christian school. In a community of 800, if you don't work there (and almost no one does) if you don't send your kids to school there (and we didn't plan to), and if you don't go to church there, you will end up knowing no one in town. Unless we exerted Herculean effort in neighborhood networking, we would be isolated; I would not even be able to get a ride to work.

Lynn had been attending a United Methodist Church in town before we were married, and I joined her. It was small in those days, with an attendance of maybe 40. We were both younger then but solid in our faith and determined to be involved. We taught Sunday schools and served on committees.

The UMC is marked by a connectional system, meaning that local parishes are "connected" to one another by belonging to the same Annual Conference. The Bishop of that Annual Conference, with the assistance of his cabinet, assigns pastors to churches where they believe there is a good fit. A pastor serves one local church for about five years, then moves on.

At one point in history, this probably made sense. But unfortunately, our experience was less than stellar. As we worked with our district superintendent to communicate the profile of pastor we needed – theologically conservative, believed in the Scriptures, embraced the centrality of Christ – we encountered pushback.

The Conference was not deaf to our concerns; it was more of a human resources problem. Relocating dozens of pastors every year within the conference and matching them up with an assignment where the salary lines up both with the pastor's expectations and the local church's budget has got to be a logistics nightmare.

The last thing they wanted from us was a refusal to accept our assigned pastor.

The next to last thing they wanted from us was a time-consuming theological discussion about what type of person we wanted in the pulpit. We had some helpful district superintendents over the years, people genuine in their faith and determined to serve our needs. But the organizational constraints were sometimes overpowering.

The problem got worse as the UMC continued slouching toward leftist politics, as Robert Bork might have put it. In 1972, at the first regular General Conference after the founding of the United Methodist Church denomination, the gay lobby presented petitions on the conference floor. The progressive motions were voted down, but at every annual conference and every four-year General (global) Conference, they kept coming back, incrementally gaining support. These efforts to recognize and affirm gays and lesbians gained traction year by year with clergy and laity.

Human sexuality was and is a lightning rod for controversy, but it was merely one of a wide range of issues dominating UMC's attention. As the leaders of the denomination embraced more liberal positions, the church mirrored the accelerating progressivism of American culture.

We, and many other congregations like ours, understood that mirroring the dominant culture was antithetical to the purpose of the church. We were determined to model ourselves more biblically. "Do not love the world, or the things in the world," says 1 John 2:15. We thought it quite likely that eventually we would be asked to accept an openly gay or lesbian pastor or youth worker.

That would be a non-starter for our people. I was confident that some gays attended church with us — How could there not be? How would we even know? Why would I even care? — and while we were called to show love and respect to them and everyone else, having one openly in the pulpit was a bridge too far.

By 2016, the fault lines between conservatives and progressives in the denomination were undeniable, and it became apparent that there would eventually be a split. In Benton, we had a new million-dollar church building. Our local congregation built it, made the down payment, and serviced the mortgage. But under UMC rules, the Conference, not the local people, owned the property.

The property control issue probably goes back 250 years to John Wesley, the founder of the Methodist movement, who wanted to maintain doctrinal purity throughout the new denomination by controlling property ownership. Those were the days when circuit riders spent hours in the saddle traveling from one church to the next, with little oversight from church leadership. But in modern times, the property ownership policy had been turned on its head. In the 21st century, it wasn't the local church that turned its back on orthodoxy; it was the leadership of the General Conference. The rank and file, especially in flyover country, remained faithful to a gospel largely untainted by politics.

In 2018, two of us met with our newly assigned pastor. This man was a good fit for us in both theology and personality. I asked him to consider how we could separate ourselves from the denomination. It was well received.

~~~~~~~~~~~~~~~~~~~~

Other Voices

Because of the politics, I had begged Curt for 30 years to let us leave the UMC. When he finally said yes, he decided to take our whole church with him. – Lynn

~~~~~~~~~~~~~~~~~~~~

One thing I believe the UMC leadership did right was to use the connectional system to assign conservative pastors to conservative churches. Ours was such a case. It turned out we had been given a pastor who had his own issues with the UMC, and he found himself with a like-minded congregation. It was a stand-up thing for the bishop and district superintendent to do, and I know they had many competing stresses during this time.

As a congregation, we had four concerns:

- We desired greater autonomy in the pastor selection process,
- We desired freedom from the UMC political environment,
- We desired to attract like-minded friends and neighbors, free from political overtones, and
- We desired an environment of scriptural accountability.

We were careful not to call out political positions with which we disagreed. It would have been frankly impossible to agree on a political platform, and anyway, we did not believe that politics was the church's primary role. It was not about any specific issue, though there were many – abortion, same-sex unions, climate change, Israel, guns, immigration, to name a few. Some of our local members disagreed with each other on many of those issues. But the fact was that the "correct" positions kept coming at us from the top down. These usually took the form of resolutions introduced at the Annual Conference and General Conference, and each local member was expected to toe the line. We were being herded toward political positions not necessarily of our choosing, and it had reached a breaking point.

In a carefully written letter, we expressed our concerns to the leadership of our Annual Conference, asking for directions on how to separate. We heard crickets chirp in response. Then, in a move that surprised us, a 2020 action taken by the General Conference gave us a path to depart the denomination ("disaffiliate") and keep our property. This was a limited offer, with the window open for three years only. No price for the building was demanded, but we were asked to pay unfunded pensions.

I reasoned that if we remained in the UMC, we would have to pay those pensions through annual appropriations. If we left, we would owe the present value of that future stream of payments. While I had serious disagreements with UMC leadership, I felt that retired pastors, staff, and other employees ought to be paid what they had been promised.

Our number came to $275,000. We paid it, some in cash and some added to the mortgage, and left the denomination, immediately establishing an independent evangelical congregation: The Benton Church... TBC.

A process for disaffiliation had been laid out by the Conference, specifying rules for a local church vote, payment terms, timelines, and commitments. We followed it scrupulously and eventually received the deed to the building, legally recorded at the county courthouse. Our official vote was something like 106 to 3. Our pastor turned in his UMC credentials, we hired him the same day, and we were on our own.

Theological Contemplations

During the writing of the U.S. Constitution, James Madison acknowledged that individuals cannot be separated from their self-interest. It will guide their actions. He established the doctrine of separation of powers within the newly designed federal government and between the states and the feds. By balancing one person's (or one department's, or one state's) self-interest against another's, he devised a system of government that he hoped would persevere. You can read about it in The Federalist Papers (*Federalist 10*).

Christians are to deny self and follow Christ, often at high personal cost. See Luke 9:23. *Whoever wants to be my disciple must deny themselves and take up their cross daily and follow me.* In the matter of leaving the emergency communications business, the temptation was confusing the noble sentiment of following Christ with the much more mundane idea of doing favors for friends.

I could have given more consideration to my own self-interest, assessing what was best for my career, family, customers, and company. This is not to be confused with selfishness. I could have fought the move, probably would have succeeded, and either Frank or Leon would have been in trouble. Perhaps a little unfortunate, but that's life in the fast lane. Realistically, they would both have landed on their feet. In the business world, similar to adopting a child, it is essential to avoid the savior mentality.

In the same way that everyone benefitted when my refund-refusing boss was fired, almost everyone would have been better off had I remained in emergency communications. (With the possible exception of the 25 service reps whose jobs I protected… there is that.) Most of us know the difference between big decisions (marriage, career, family, location) and little decisions (which restaurant, leisure time, buy the Ford or buy the Chevy). The big decision I confronted was a matter of career direction and deserved more thought than I gave it. It was also a gold-plated opportunity to ask advice from senior managers where I worked. *In the multitude of counselors there is safety,* says Proverbs 11:14 (KJV). But I did not ask.

It's over and done with, but the experience is not without value. I cannot go back to 1998 and do it over; no one is owed an apology and there is no restitution to make. So, I draw this lesson: When one finds oneself internally flogged for a decision like this, where there is no recourse, the feeling one experiences is not conviction by the Holy Spirit; it is temptation by the devil.

Condemning oneself for past decisions like this can be debilitating regarding self-confidence, which is the critical component of success in career progression and interpersonal relationships. The popular targets of self-recrimination are: *Did I marry the wrong person? Did I go to the wrong college (or not go to college)? Did I start the wrong career?*

Twenty years on, none can be changed, and no one is owed an apology. I believe these are favorite tools of the devil to keep one from following God's leading. The devil is merely a deceiver. He cannot actually do anything to us. That's why Psalm 23 talks of "the valley of the *shadow* of death" rather than "the valley of death."

The threat of death is also a mere shadow. When the real thing comes, you'll probably know it.

*****

What was different about protecting the jobs of 25 service reps on the one hand and protecting the jobs of my two buddies on the other hand? Good question, but there was a substantive distinction. I had no organizational responsibility to Frank and Leon; their careers were their own. They were both quite capable of using internal company contacts to find different positions or, as actually came about, to separate from the company entirely. Besides that, there was only one of them in jeopardy. It's easier to find one position for a manager with a wide range of experience than 25 positions for people with a limited skill set, regardless of how competent they might be.

Also, the service reps had few internal political associations that could help them. And most importantly, they were my people; I was their unit manager and had, I believed, a moral responsibility to keep them employed, if possible. The choice of the Billing Inquiry Unit was a poor alternative for them but much better than the humiliation of a surplus, which would have meant permanent separation from the company.

The stress I inflicted on my staff friend Jim was entirely appropriate. He was a competent and thoughtful second-line manager engaged in a successful career. I had no problem asking him to step up and solve the problem, just as I was doing. *From everyone who has been given much, much will be demanded; and from the one who has been entrusted with much, much more will be asked (Luke 12:48).*

While the two situations looked similar, they were quite different. I succeeded with one while falling somewhat short with the other.

Of course, everyone fails sometime at something. Only of Jesus could it be said, "He has done everything well." *(Mark 7:37).*

One could argue He had a leg up on the rest of us. (A friend of mine, an attorney by day and a superb ad-lib jazz trumpet player by night, once opined, "In jazz, there is no such thing as wrong notes, only poor choices.") If there is no actual sin involved, no forgiveness to ask, and no restitution to make, how can one come to terms with the sense of failure?

As with anything else, we find healing and restoration in Scripture. I have found passages like Jeremiah 10:23 helpful in acknowledging that while we are indeed responsible for planning and executing wisely, God is the One Who leads. *Lord, I know that people's lives are not their own; it is not for them to direct their steps.*

Lynn and I attended a Christian seminar once in the 1980s. It stretched over several days and covered many issues, one of them how to deal with personal failure. The metaphor used was of a jeweler chipping away the dross from a diamond in the rough. The jeweler's job was to wield a tiny hammer and chisel; the diamond's job was to stay locked in the vise without moving. When the diamond attempted to squirm away from the impact, the chisel could cut deeper than intended and remove too much material.

However, the illustration went that a characteristic of the diamond is that it always retains the same crystalline structure, whether large or small. So, when the impact does its unintended violence, there remains a perfect diamond; it's just smaller than before.

Then, when a jewelry set is created, the jeweler must select both big and little diamonds. Both have their place, and without both, the setting loses attractiveness. Did I make a "poor choice" somewhere that altered the trajectory of my life? Probably so; it happens all the time. But by the grace of God, I remain instrumental.

This was a hugely influential insight for me, and one I have returned to many times, probably because my litany of failures is strong, robust, and ever-growing.

*****

When I sensed the time was right to retire, I returned to Colossians 3:23–24 again and again: *Whatever you do, work at it with all your heart, as working for the Lord, not for human masters... It is the Lord Christ you are serving.*

I determined that I would remain active and engaged up to the end, and I set expectations with customers with whom I was close so they were not left high and dry. During the last few months at work, I was able to close out all the gnarly projects I had taken on so as not to make someone else decipher my work. I could almost hear it: *"What the heck was Curt thinking when he started that???"*

I had a mental picture of a Navy carrier aircraft on takeoff, accelerating off the end of the deck.

*****

The church thing: Realistically, there was every reason to suspect that our disaffiliation effort would fail, but from the beginning, I presented the public conviction that TBC would separate from the UMC and retain ownership of the property. I communicated this to my peers on the Futures team appointed to explore whether and how to disaffiliate. My conviction was perhaps without basis, but I continued to assert success: "Gang, this is going to happen. We just have to figure out how and then make it work."

I was committed to it, and having sent the letter to the bishop, I had put a stake in the ground: We are separating, one way or the other. So, the decision was made at that point; afterward, it was just a matter of remaining consistent with that commitment.

This was a forerunner to that resolution (the working hypothesis) I promised myself after the cancer diagnosis. "I am the toughest hombre in this ward" was not philosophically too distant from "Gang, this is going to happen," nor from "Make it happen, Jim. We are going to do this." The disaffiliation process – filled with conflict, uncertainty, doubt, and hard work – was a training ground.

But then everything is, and the next hill is always taller than the previous one. Intellectually, I could recognize this concept, but in practice, I had no idea how incredibly unscalable that next one would be.

Chapter 5

Normandy, France, 1944

Early on the morning of June 6, 1944, 225 soldiers of the 2nd Ranger Battalion, U.S. Army, commanded by Lt. Colonel James E. Rudder, boarded nine landing craft and headed for Pointe du Hoc on the Normandy Coast, situated at the junction of Utah and Omaha beaches. Their mission was to neutralize six 155 mm guns the Germans had placed in this critically strategic position. On high ground, they could be used to oppose the Allied D-Day landings on both beaches. "Rudder's Rangers" were supported by the 5th Ranger Battalion that was to come ashore a half hour after the initial assault. *(www.armyhistory.org)*

High winds and choppy seas drove the landing craft off course; they made landfall under heavy enemy fire several hundred yards from their planned landing point. As a result, they were 40 minutes behind schedule. One boat was swamped in the surf, capsized, and all occupants lost. Among them was the official news reporter; he and his camera gear were lost, which is why very few photos, and no video footage of the attack, exist.

Rudder's Rangers commenced what they believed was a suicide mission scaling a hundred-foot cliff using rocket-propelled grappling hooks with rope ladders attached. From above, enemy soldiers opposed them with small arms fire and hand grenades. Seaspray made some ropes too heavy for the missiles to lift and too slippery to climb; mud made uniforms and hands slick.

However, some of the assault force made it to the top and engaged the German defenders, who began to retreat. (The .30-06 American Browning Automatic Rifle – "BAR" – was a game changer, with its full auto rate of fire at 400 rounds per minute.)

Establishing a small "beachhead" on the clifftop, the Rangers were bewildered to find the big guns had been moved. The original heavy German concrete installations housed dummy guns made of utility poles.

An hour after landing, with the battle still raging, a two-man Ranger patrol discovered the camouflaged guns unattended 250 yards inland. They spiked the guns with thermite grenades, disabling them.

Mission accomplished, but at an enormous cost. By the following morning, only 100 of the original 225 soldiers remained fit for duty. Most of the rest lie in the American Cemetery at Colleville-sur-Mer. These were the men President Ronald Reagan lauded as "the boys of Pointe du Hoc" in his D-Day 40th-anniversary speech delivered from that Normandy Coast location.

Did they believe they would succeed? Yes and no. While most soldiers were convinced that they would die or be severely wounded in the attack – and they were right – they believed the assault would succeed. What drove them forward? Beyond the rarely spoken conviction that freedom was somehow worth their sacrifice, it was probably nothing more than they had voluntarily determined, "This will I do." That, and the expectations of their comrades.

While we do not typically wage our battles with guns and bullets – although, thankfully, some do on our behalf – the conviction is the same. "I am the toughest person in this cancer ward," is brother to, "This will I do."

PART II: THE CANCER WARD

Chapter 6

Caring Bridge Journal, June 24 – June 26, 2022

June 24

This site has been created to help the many folks that care about both Curt and the Ghormley family keep abreast of how Curt is doing.

This Wednesday, Curt went in for a routine annual physical. Later that day, the office called him and instructed him to go to the ER immediately. Andover Medical Center diagnosed him with Acute Leukemia, and sent him to St. Francis where he is currently.

To date, he has had blood transfusions and he starts chemotherapy today.

As more details and updates come available, we will make them available here. Of course, much thanks for the outpouring of prayers and support on behalf of the Ghormley family.

June 25

Chemo Day 1. Very much appreciate all the prayers and your kind words. Leukemia,,, whooda thunk it? They got the cardio readings yesterday so they can mix the proper chemo brew. It should start this afternoon.

Ephesians 5;20 Giving thanks always for all things unto God and the Father in the name of our Lord Jesus Christ. Curt

June 25

Chemo Day 1 suppl. The first 3 days of this 7 day regimen include 2 different cocktails, both strong but one of them (the red one, administered with the large grease gun) quite aggressive. The latter 4 days only the milder fellow is continued. After about 8 hours of this today I don't feel any different… still my upbeat, impatient and slightly cynical self. But I sense a cloud bank forming. Kids came in for a visit, very good to see them. Stay in the game! Curt

June 26

Chemo Day 2. Ready for round 2. Of the 2 cocktails, the more mild brew drips for 24 hours while the stout fellow only works 8 hour shifts. Both are fairly nasty, as they must be, in order to kill off all the cells you normally depend on for various protections. Once all the protective troops are out of the way the bone marrow will produce a new crop, hopefully with behavior conducive to a more harmonious outcome. Or so says the brochure.

Psalm 53:5 There were they in great fear, where no fear was.

Chin up! Curt

June 26

Chemo Day 2 suppl. Pretty lethargic this morning, which was to be expected. I managed to choke down all the meals, none of which I had appetite for, lest Nurse Ratchet would put me on The List. Did 2 (short) laps in the hallway with Caleb and David (sons who showed up wondering about the will), and managed some modest success with bodily operations you can guess at. I'm exhausted. This is harder than tent camping. End Day 2. Smile/grimace emoji. Curt

Inflection Point 1 – You Do Not Have Two Weeks

When the doctor's office calls two hours after a routine annual wellness exam, it's generally not a good sign. With urgency in her voice, the nurse said, "Please go immediately to an ER and ask them to repeat the blood test. Your platelets should be at 150, and they are at 4."

At work, I scanned the list of emails awaiting my urgent attention. "Four *what?*" I asked.

She replied, "It's just a measure, don't worry about the number. But please have the blood test repeated as soon as possible. Like right now, please." I told her I would and hung up, wondering if this would take long. I had already presumed on my schedule by coming to work late that morning, and this test would constitute my lunch hour. I would be obligated to take some vacation time if it went longer.

Chapter 6

The day had started typically. I met with Tyler for breakfast at 6:15 a.m., our usual Wednesday morning routine, for Scripture memory review. He was working through The Navigator's New Topical Memory System (TMS), 60 verses on 30 different topics, and had asked for my help. I had memorized the TMS 50 years earlier and had always told anyone who would listen (a short list when discussing Scripture memory) that learning Bible verses on your own is impossible. You must have another person to whom you can recite the passage out loud and who can correct you as needed. Tyler called my bluff, asked for my help, and proved to be an excellent student.

After breakfast, I saw my primary care physician (PCP) for a routine annual checkup. Not that I needed it, being a poster boy for health and vitality even at the ripe age of 68. Sometimes I blow off the physical, but this year I decided to do it because of another minor bacterial infection that was active and for which I had seen a urologist the day before. For 15 years, I had been afflicted two or three times a year with what the doctors concluded must be cellulitis. This involved a sudden swelling of what I shall delicately refer to as the nether regions, which they believed was caused by bacteria lodging in scar tissue left over from hernia surgeries.

Whatever. We all have our baggage. I called it the Long Beach Flu because that was where I was when it first appeared. Which made for an interesting road trip, but that's for another time.

This time the swelling had gone high and had not receded within a week, as I was accustomed, ergo the visit to the urologist.

In a manner of speaking, the urologist is a hardware guy. His initial suggestion was to remove the offending body part, which in this case was Mr. Lefty. This made me stare off into space for a moment. Then I told him that might be okay… I guessed… but wondered if there might not be a software solution (e.g., drugs) that should be explored before we resorted to the knife. He seemed disappointed but acquiesced and scheduled a sonogram for two weeks out.

At the PCP annual the following day, the doc and I discussed my overall health, the urologist visit, right-wing politics, a meddlesome federal government, and the deplorable state of Young Persons Who Do Not Understand Civic Responsibility – all the usual topics he and I explore. Then, he turned me over to a nurse who drew blood and asked me to fill a small cup.

While attempting to execute the latter, I became aware that the gauze pad at the blood extraction site was soaked bright red. Blood was running down my arm, and my shirt was becoming soaked. Being a farm boy with a college education, I'm no dummy; I can recognize unusual when I see it. When I emerged from the bathroom, the fill-the-cup routine forgotten, the nurse blanched and whisked me out of the reception area. Wide-eyed patients suddenly wondered if they should have seen a different sawbones. The nurse wrapped my arm and sent me on my way.

I went to work. At the time, I was a road sales rep for a small Wichita business selling meat processing equipment. As pointed out, I had retired from a 36-year career with a communications technology company. I bought and dabbled in my own firewood business for a few years; immensely entertaining and great for my health and fitness but financially desultory.

Eventually, I decided to quit being a drag anchor on the economy and return to work. This small company took pity on me and offered me a sales territory in Pennsylvania and New England, handling it remotely from Wichita. (It makes perfect sense, I know.) I flew one week a month and used my silver-tongued oratorical skills to convince customers that a family-owned business 1,500 miles away is more responsive to their needs than the major supplier a hundred miles down the road. Which we are, and in which we take well-deserved pride. It's a quality outfit, and I am honored to be part of it.

Chapter 6

At about 11:00 a.m., the nurse called with the aforementioned urgent message. I drove to an emergency room close to home, checked in, explained the situation, and asked for a blood test. In a few minutes, they had me in a bed with an intravenous drip, and there seemed to be more activity than warranted.

Eventually, it occurred to me that I probably should call Lynn to let her know I was at an ER for a blood test. I assured her it was nothing serious (because nothing serious ever happens to me) and there was no reason for her to come. She took it in stride, as is her wont. She does not scare easily.

A few minutes later, a doctor was explaining the difference between lymphoma and leukemia.

"I'm sorry, I missed something here," I said, perplexed. "Why are we talking about these L-words?"

"Because your blood counts are way off," he explained patiently. "Your platelets are at two, where you say they were at four earlier today. They are nose-diving. Your hemoglobin is low, and your white blood cells are low."

"That's bad?"

"Actually," he said flatly, "that's leukemia."

There followed what we might call a pregnant pause. I could hear the hum of air conditioning and the indistinct murmur of voices from the next room. I broke the silence. "Is that a diagnosis?"

"No, of course not. We're just an ER. We're not qualified to make that diagnosis." He raised an eyebrow and nodded confidently. "But when whites are low, hemoglobin is low, and platelets are low, that's leukemia."

So, there it was. The stars had aligned, and I was the winner. This could be a long lunch hour. Lynn called to see if I had gone back to work yet. Well, I said, not exactly. I invited her to the ER and advised her that I had left my pickup in the south parking lot.

That night I was transported to Ascension St. Francis Hospital in Wichita, which sports a fully functional state-of-the-art Cancer Center. I was deposited in a private room with my cell phone, no charger and spotty Wi-Fi coverage. I was left to contemplate many things, foremost among them how to spell leukemia. That was Day 1 of hospitalization, and I had no idea it would stretch into nearly three months.

~~~~~~~~~~~~~~~~~~~~

Other Voices

The day was unremarkable: Dishes, laundry, planning dinner. Being June, I might have been deciding on whether to fish, kayak, or bike in the afternoon. Curt called about 1:00 to say he was at the hospital. He had a routine check-up that morning, and a nurse had called asking him to repeat some tests.

Later, I called Curt thinking he had probably gone back to work. Unexpectedly, he said, "Maybe you'd better come down here." The rest of this day and the next 82 were extraordinary. Extraordinary people, procedures, and medicines. Extraordinary machines, facilities, and care. And above all, an extraordinary God who attended us and still does. – Lynn

~~~~~~~~~~~~~~~~~~~~

June 23 The following day began the doctor meetings. There was a dizzying array of them and were generally grouped into five categories for my case: Oncology, Infectious Disease, Nephrology (kidneys), Cardiac, and the Hospitalist who is to understand what the other four are doing and communicate to the customer. (And don't forget the surgical team, who gave the impression of sharpening scalpels expectantly and hoping for The Call.) It being summer, every doctor had vacation time to burn, so an associate substituted for the principal. The substitutes also had vacation time, so more associates were introduced.

I learned that, in general, I would see each doctor discipline every day, making five random visits daily from a pool of potentially 38 different doctors and assistants. They were from Lebanon, Syria, Ukraine, Vietnam, India, Jordan, Kenya, Pakistan. Most were U.S. citizens, with a few on work visas. We even had a couple of token native-born North Americans. What a great country this is!

The doctor consultations were interspersed with other activities: A nurse taking vital signs every four hours *(Me: "Can't you just enter the previous dope again? It can't be that different." Nurse: "Not a chance!")*, another nurse explaining each IV and oral med, and a seemingly never-ending supply of experts.

There was a pharmacy specialist explaining why this drug and not that drug, a housekeeper in and out cleaning the bathroom, sweeping the floor, taking out the trash, an administrative case worker explaining insurance coverages, a chaplain to ensure my spiritual well-being... and I concluded early on that cancer is not a lazy man's disease. Something is happening all the time. All this, and try to write a clever and engaging Caring Bridge post every day.

Caring Bridge? It is a Godsend. Caring Bridge dot org is a free website, Facebook-like, where I can post a journal entry describing today's health status. Those who log onto the site can make comments, others may comment on their comment, and so on. Those who wish can post a message and a donation to the "Tribute" section; this keeps CB in business. CB keeps me from receiving 50 texts daily from well-intentioned friends who want to know how I'm doing. *(I have a terminal disease and may not last the summer. How you doin'?)* They can just read my daily post. During this ordeal, I collected about 250 regular followers. Most of these are from my local church, but there are also people from my work, City Council, my high school graduating class, and other activities Lynn and I are involved in.

So, we were off and running. It was still a little perplexing to me, and I had not yet had time to process what leukemia meant for me. I knew it was cancer, that cancer killed people, and that usually there was some lengthy and uncomfortable treatment regimen between diagnosis and death. That did not sound at all appealing, but I knew enough to know I didn't know enough... I needed to discuss it with the oncologist.

June 24 Early that second day between doctors, I called Jeffrey, one of the more accomplished Information Technologists I know. I asked him to set up a Caring Bridge site using my wife's credentials. He contacted Lynn an hour later to advise that the site was ready for prime time, and I posted the first journal entry.

~~~~~~~~~~~~~~~~~~~~
Other Voices

When your maybe-going-to-die-soon-but-also-maybe-not Sunday School teacher of nearly three decades sends a text asking if you can talk, you say yes. I don't remember the specifics of our call, mostly pacing in my bedroom half-dressed for work, learning about blood cells. And me getting far too sappy... I think I even said "I love you" which was completely uncalled for.

I was asked to sort out a communications hub, which was easy enough thanks to the interface available. At the time I didn't appreciate just how important that platform would prove to be for all of us... Curt's daily posts and the praying community following along for the next three months. – Jeffrey

~~~~~~~~~~~~~~~~~~~~

Chapter 6

The initial conversation with the oncologist would be the first inflection point in this journey: A turning point where only bad options presented themselves. Each option carried a high risk of... an undesirable outcome. In other words, death. There would eventually be six inflection points. By the time we were done, this had all the earmarks of a multi-level computer game, except without do-overs. The first time the screen turned red, it would be lights out.

*****

That night about 10:00 p.m., I was visited by a pair of technicians – the Sam and Dan show – who installed a PICC line. (Peripherally Inserted Central Catheter.)

The line went into my right bicep. It was a tube 16 inches long that somehow found its way magically along a vein (the superior *vena cava*, I was told) to a place near the heart. There were three tubes, each with an access port, encased inside a single shell dangling near my armpit. This way, drugs could be pushed into the body while extracting blood as needed.

The PICC also protects the veins from the poison of chemotherapy drugs. Before PICCs were in everyday use, cancer patients receiving the very potent drip of Idarubicin (on which more later) experienced redness and chafing.

This was like a bad sunburn along the skin surface over the vein used. The standard explanation doctors offered patients was that this was merely part of the chemo process; sorry that it's uncomfortable, but we are trying to keep you alive here.

The advent of the PICC insulated the vein from the drug and removed this discomfort. Who thinks this stuff up?

~~~~~~~~~~~~~~~~~~~~~
Other Voices

Curt messaged me at 5:00 a.m. that first morning. Then, others began texting to prepare me. I think that's what scared me most. I knew it was bad and that I couldn't get to him. I finally got my head in the game and asked myself the question Curt had always asked: What does God's Word say? So, I grimaced, opened it up, found Philippians 1:21 (to live is Christ and to die is gain)... and found my solid ground, although I didn't like it one bit. I didn't want to blubber anymore; I just wanted to keep him company. I thanked God for technology and began sending him video messages. – Charity

~~~~~~~~~~~~~~~~~~~~~

Sam and Dan were nothing short of impressive. One was older, no doubt the team leader, and he kept up a running commentary from my left side, while the younger fellow did all the work on my right arm.

They built a plastic screen around the site. I could not see exactly what was happening – the barrier was to keep me from infecting the site with breath, sneeze, or cough – and they also masked me. They were scrupulously clean. I knew the purpose of the commentary was to distract me from the activity, and I did not object, but I would have been interested in seeing the operation. I'll have to wait for the movie.

It took some time to do. It was midnight before the procedure was finished. Now I had a semi-permanent pathway for drugs. This was a beneficial alternative to stabbing a vein in my hand or arm every time another IV was set up. The number of IV drips would become legion.

But all of that was merely background to the big project – establishing the leukemia treatment plan.

Chapter 6

June 25 The oncologist, Doctor N, was from Lebanon and shared the same last name as the urologist I had seen two days before. They were cousins. I suggested this was a ruse to defeat malpractice, as in: "Oh no, that wasn't me; that was my cousin. Have your attorney contact him; it's a common error." He took it good-naturedly and enjoyed the humor. But that was hardly the point of our first visit.

He came to my hospital room and sat opposite the bed in a straight-backed chair, leaning forward. "You should know," he said, "that most patients who come to me with numbers like yours do not survive to walk out." That comment has a marvelous way of compelling one's attention; he had mine entirely.

"But there are things we can do," he continued, "to improve your chances. First, you have this collateral condition of swelling. We will put you on an aggressive regimen of antibiotics for two weeks to solve that problem in the short term. Then we will move to chemotherapy to treat the leukemia."

"That would be good," I replied. "I am ready for the swelling to go away."

"We'll do that," he said with a nod. "Let me review the case notes so far, and I will get back to you."

I felt better after this. The doctor seemed assertive and honest, a straight shooter with no spin. I found out just how straight two hours later.

*****

Fortunately, Lynn had brought me the phone charger, so while the doctor was gone, I researched what I could on leukemia. It was enlightening but not especially encouraging.

Acute Myeloid Leukemia (AML) strikes older Americans at an average age of 68. So far, so good; I was apparently in the sweet spot. "Myeloid" refers to the type of cells the cancer attacks. The "acute" word in the title means it is exceptionally aggressive.

CLL Society dot org lists the different types of leukemia, all sharing standard 3-letter abbreviations. The first letter, "A," references Acute; "C" in that position indicates Chronic. The third letter is always "L" for Leukemia. The letter in the middle distinguishes what leukemia attacks. The Acutes include AML (Acute Myeloid Leukemia) and ALL (Acute Lymphoblastic Leukemia).

Leukemia attacks the manufacturing process of the bone marrow. Myeloid (or myelogenous) Leukemia develops when the marrow starts producing immature blood cells, sometimes called myeloblasts. Lymphoblastic (aka, lymphocytic) Leukemia develops when abnormal white blood cells accumulate in the marrow and divide rapidly. They crowd out healthy whites.

In the Chronic category, there is CLL (Chronic Lymphocytic Leukemia) and CML (Chronic Myeloid Leukemia). The Lymphocytic type grows defective cells slowly, and at a certain point, they travel into the bloodstream and crowd out the healthy versions. This is the type most associated with the kids you see in TV commercials.

CML is similar but is characterized by a "Philadelphia chromosome" formed when chunks of chromosomes 22 and 9 break away from their natural host points and trade places. *(Cancercenter.com)* Makes perfect sense, no?

How do the chromosomes know to do this? And why? I have long suspected nothing good comes from Philadelphia. Except for the Declaration and Constitution, and Bill of Rights. And maybe Rocky Balboa. But not much else.

Chapter 6

One site suggested that the three-month survival rate for newly diagnosed AML cases was 27 percent. Not an especially sanguine outlook. *Statistics, schmatistics.*

*****

Doctor N reappeared in my room and took his chair. He was accompanied by Doctor A, the infectious disease specialist whose job it was to manage the antibiotics.

"I have concluded my first thought was a poor choice," began Doctor N. "We both would like to have you on a strong course of antibiotics for two weeks before beginning chemo." Doctor A nodded her agreement. "But there is a problem." He paused and the two medicos exchanged a look. He returned his gaze to me.

"You do not have two weeks. We are going to start chemotherapy immediately." The statement hung in the air.

You do not have two weeks. My remaining life span had just gone from 20 years to 14 days. All righty, then.

"Are we still doing the antibiotics?" I asked.

"Yes, we are," replied Doctor A. "Lots of antibiotics. But we will administer the chemotherapy at the same time."

"Won't they fight against each other?"

"Yes, they will," Doctor N assured me, "but don't worry. The chemo is a schoolyard bully and will win that contest. But some of the antibiotics will survive and provide whatever protection they can. We will begin both tomorrow morning."

This interchange, with both doctors present, showed me beyond question that the oncologist, Doctor N, was calling the shots. The infection may be a problem, but if we didn't deal with the leukemia, nothing else would matter.

And then, of course, we did not actually begin chemotherapy the following morning. The antibiotics, yes; the chemo, no. Logistics intervened.

The chemotherapy is a unique brew, a cocktail of various ingredients made from a basic formula and then tailored to each person as needed. Before legally administering the standard mixture, they must determine whether there will be unexpected damage to the patient, specifically to his heart. For this, an EKG is required.

A technician showed up in my room, EKG cart in tow. Attaching a dozen leads to my chest took five minutes; collecting the results took 30 seconds. Removing the leads (and a substantial quantity of hair – don't worry, it's all disappearing soon anyway) took another five minutes, and she was gone. But the EKG had to be read, interpreted, and sent to the chemotherapy cocktail lab. This process occupied the rest of the day, and the lab only worked until 4:00 p.m. This makes sense because they probably start their day at 4:00 a.m. to prepare for their patients.

Also, the cocktail lab at St. Francis was offline for remodeling, so we had to use the lab at St. Joseph Hospital, across town. St. Joseph received the EKG results at 4:30 p.m. (when no one was there to accept it), and the next day they prepared the cocktail and sent it by courier to St. Francis. It has a short shelf life, so time is of the essence once brewed.

So far, we had run two days off the clock, and I recalled something important about 14 days… but I was unable to influence the timetable, and I sensed that complaining to the nursing staff (who held my life by a slender thread) would perhaps be counterproductive. I'm sure the doctor was quite frustrated by these delays, but to his credit, he acted as though all was working according to plan.

Chapter 6

So, in less than a week, I went from a robust, healthy, highly experienced sales rep, energetically growing a virgin New England market among butchers and slaughterhouses, to a bed-ridden senior citizen with two weeks to live. My, how things change. I reasoned that once we were done with the chemotherapy, a prospect fraught with uncertainty and probably considerable discomfort – *yeah, so what?* – I could get back to work. It should take about a month.

Think again.

Theological Contemplations

It never happens until it happens. The unexpected blood-soaked gauze where the lab sample had been taken, followed by the call from the nurse, proved the insight of Psalm 32:6. *Let all the faithful pray to you while you may be found; surely the rising of the mighty waters will not reach them.*

My dad was not a particularly spiritual man. Like most men of his generation, he did not speak freely of his faith, but one comment I recall frequently came up*: Be on speakin' terms with the Lord.* By which he meant: *Pray while He may be found; make a habit of routine prayer; keep your accounts short; don't let yourself get caught short when sudden disaster strikes.* This was surprising wisdom from a Navy Chief, or maybe that was where he learned it.

*****

At this point in my life, I had for near-on 50 years practiced a daily devotional time – Quiet Time, I called it – involving short Bible reading and a brief prayer. It's not much, but a 20-minute session early every morning became a habit and seemed to set the needle for the day's activities. I do not expect to find a nugget every day that purifies my thoughts for hours. My recall of the passage is frequently forgotten as my mind is overcome with events.

But the following day, I am back at it again, and sometimes a few highlights stick with me.

Consider the surprise that ambushed King Hezekiah in Isaiah 36. Sennacherib, the king of Assyria, sent his field commander to lay siege to Jerusalem, where Hezekiah reigned over Judah. The message posed a daunting rhetorical question: *Do not let Hezekiah mislead you when he says, 'The Lord will deliver us.' Have the gods of any nations ever delivered their lands from the hand of the king of Assyria? (Isaiah 36:18)*

After some back and forth between the siege force and the Jerusalem defenders, a letter was delivered with Sennacherib's ultimatum. Seeing what Hezekiah did with that letter offers a path for us when we receive bad news.

*Hezekiah received the letter from the messengers and read it. Then he went up to the temple of the Lord and spread it out before the Lord. And Hezekiah prayed to the Lord: "Lord Almighty, the God of Israel, enthroned between the cherubim, **you alone are God** over all the kingdoms of the earth. You have made heaven and earth. Give ear, Lord, and hear; open your eyes, Lord, and see; listen to all the words Sennacherib has sent to ridicule the living God. **It is true**, Lord, that the Assyrian kings have laid waste all these peoples and their lands. They have thrown their gods into the fire and destroyed them, for they were not gods but only wood and stone, fashioned by human hands. Now, Lord our God, **deliver us from his hand**, so that all the kingdoms of the earth may know that you, Lord, are the only God." Isaiah 37:14-20 (emphasis added).*

In receiving the letter, reading it, and opening it before the Lord, the outline is clear:

He **acknowledged** God's sovereignty – *You alone are God over all the kingdoms of the earth (vs. 16)*

He **assented** to the facts on the ground – *It is true, Lord, that the Assyrian kings have laid waste all these peoples and their lands (vs. 18)*

He **asked** for God's intervention – *Now, Lord our God, deliver us from his hand (vs. 20)*

Chapter 6

This pattern can be followed when we get bad news: A grade report, a letter from the bank, a notice from the attorney, a collection letter from an agency, a goodbye note from a partner. Even lab results from the doctor.

Acknowledge that God is sovereign; assent to – do not deny – the truth of the situation; ask God to show the right way to respond.

I found that it especially applies when the doctor says, "You do not have two weeks."

San Diego, 1943

One day Dad ran into a fellow Chief Petty Officer who had a deep scar down the side of his hairline, above the ear. "Where'd you pick that up?" Dad asked.

The chief explained he had served on a destroyer during the landing on Tarawa, the first large-scale Marine beachhead of the war. The tides were unpredictable, and that morning the sea uncovered a coral reef some 500 yards offshore, usually concealed just beneath the waves. The landing craft, loaded with Marines, would have to contend with that reef on their way to the beach.

It was an opposed landing – Japanese defenders brought the Marines under heavy machine gun and artillery fire – and the tide happened to be low, unbeknownst to the Americans. The reef was submerged under barely 18 inches of water and, in some places, exposed entirely. The landing craft had a three-foot draft.

As dozens of landing craft got hung up on the reef, the chief explained, shells began to explode among them. The Japanese knew perfectly well where the reef was and had already registered their weapons at that distance. Machine gun fire raked the invaders.

"The Old Man got on the P.A.," the chief continued, referring to the ship's captain. "He said, 'I want a chief and a Bosun's Mate in each motor launch. Go in and get those Marines; either take them into shore or bring them back here. But get them out of there!' So, I jumped into a boat with a sailor, and we headed for the reef."

"And the scar?" Dad asked.

"After we got those guys into the launch with their equipment and delivered them to the beach, I finally figured out what was getting in my eyes. There was blood all over my face. I took a round along the side of my head, right above my ear."

"Where was your tin hat?" Dad wanted to know.

"Back In my quarters below-decks, of course," the chief said. "We were five miles offshore and the last thing I needed was a helmet."

That's all I have of their conversation. One can only wonder – in awe – at the prospect of two sailors struggling to get 40 Marines with weapons and packs across the gunwale into a wooden motorboat under relentless artillery and machine gun fire. Then driving a quarter mile into that fire, and doing this repeatedly, to deliver sodden men to the beach until the job was done.

We do not always get to choose the trials we face; only how we face them.

Chapter 7

Caring Bridge Journal, June 27 – July 14, 2022

June 27

Chemo Day 3. This is the 3rd of 3 chances for the strong and brave-hearted cocktail to do his best against the wicked red blood/white blood traitors. Which means tomorrow I should begin to feel the battle… internally. Still 4 more days of the milder juice. Somewhat milder, but you wouldn't want to meet him in a dark alley without a capable nurse, of whom we seem to have a plethora. I slept deep between insistent awakenings, and it appears I have gained some 43 lbs since Wednesday, testament to said nursing staff with electronic hoses, a first-world PICC line, and an unlimited supply of Medicare-funded bags of who knows what. Don't get between them and their liquids.

Psalm 91:5-6. Thou shalt not be afraid for the terror by night, nor for the arrow that flieth by day, nor for the pestilence that walketh in darkness…

It's a new perspective on liquid courage. Stay the course! Curt

June 28

Chemo Day 4 suppl. Well, I'm exhausted, how about you? Lynn helped me with hallway laps, and while the floor plan is confusing there are copious signs to tell you where you are. They give little clue about how to get somewhere else, however. "So now I am at room 71XX. Which way is room 73XX?" Well duh, that would be in the 7-3 hallway, now wouldn't it? It's just past Family Room D, around the corner from Family Room 3, and which is near the snack machine where the power drinks don't work.

And so on.

This was supposed to be the hard day for chemotherapy we always hear about - nasty symptoms and all - but it's been generally easy. But there is always tomorrow.

White blood cell count was at 0.1 this morning, headed for 0.0 by Friday. A week from Saturday (maybe Chemo 14, but that could change) we will do the bone marrow biopsy to assess percent that is composed of blast cells. (Blast cells are bad.). There is a max percent they will accept to declare the marrow is cooperating in the development of good white cells.

I say "we" are going to do the biopsy; actually, I think one party is to do the drilling and extraction and the other is to lie there in a state of extreme discomfort for an uncertain yet interminable period of time. I understand you may have a choice of broomstick handles to bite upon. That would be a plus. We'll take 'em where we can get 'em.

Enjoy your evening! Curt

June 30

Chemo Day 6. The days never really end here, what with vital signs required every 4 hours. So I bounced out of bed, sort of, at 600a today, made myself mobile with the portable juice bar tree, and performed morning ablutions standing at the sink. Independence feels great!

I went for a cheerful walk in the hallway, sporting the green plaid Chemo kilt this time, spreading joy and good cheer among grumpy-looking people. Wassup? You guys all sick, or what?

I ordered breakfast and wolfed it down, oatmeal, biscuit, 2 scram, bacon; then took another fast hallway lap. And barely made it back to the room before I collapsed Into bed exhausted. Slept for 2 hours.

Somebody must've spiked the OJ.

Hebrews 2:14 And deliver them who through fear of death were all their lifetime subject to bondage.

Once I wake up maybe I can write more.

Zzzzzz…. Curt

July 02

Chemo Day 8. Okay… let's all try to keep up. The hospital stay began 3 days before Hospitalization and started on night 22 June. My Chemo Day [n] reports relate to what they say- Chemo days - bc that is how the doctors plan and schedule treatments. Lynn's hospitalization status reports are based on the entire length of the incarceration.

Just thot you should hear that now, while the drugs have prompted a slight bit of lucidity.

I will continue to publish Chemo Day reports, even though chemotherapy is now over, because there are other milestones to come; they will be identified on the calendar with reference to the beginning of chemo. (Example: bone marrow biopsy on Chemo Day 14). There will be tests, biopsies, scans, procedures, and anything else necessary for adequate asset depreciation and for satisfying Master Purchase Agreement pharmaceutical terms and conditions. But I see I have become crassly commercial again.

Philippians 1:20 According to my earnest expectation and my hope, that in nothing I shall be ashamed, but that with all boldness, as always, so now also Christ shall be magnified in my body, whether it be by life, or by death.

Chapter 7

Anyway, painkillers are good, anti-nausea is good, nurses are outstanding, and this vanilla protein shake is to die for. Curt

July 02

Chemo Day 7 suppl. (Fri 1 Jul). Sleep sleep sleep; take it where you can get it. I think I lost the entire day in bed. Last night I asked for a feel good pill to calm me. Have never done one before but I was stir crazy in the blankets and ready to make a break for it, which would be inadvisable.

Sores in the mouth are worse, inhibit swallowing, but they make a mean protein shake here, chocolate peanut butter.

So... no visitors (but let Lynn decide). I can barely talk and feel that charades would not be dignified. C

July 03

Chemo Day 9. Another day, another protein shake. I slept well last night till about 100am, then read for a while and watched Frazier re-runs.

Drugs: My sense is that pharmaceutical drug regimens have improved so much in the last 10 years that anything I thought I knew about chemotherapy has been rendered irrelevant. And I am glad it has.

Staff: I don't know how you would find a hospital staff more competent, dedicated or engaged than this one. From the oncologist to the house cleaner they are all "All-In." Two of the house cleaners prayed over me yesterday, impromptu; and not just prayed: this was Jesus-exalting, Full Gospel, victorious praise and petition.

The Crash: and which I am told we are in the middle of it now. Pain, discomfort, boredom... you'd think the guy was sick.

Romans 8:15 For ye have not received the spirit of bondage again to fear; but ye have received the Spirit of adoption, whereby we cry, Abba, Father.

I am wearing my camo chemo kilt today, but there is not a good way to photograph it without embarrassing all of us. Thank you Rita!

Enjoy church today! This is the day that the Lord hath made. Curt

July 03

Chemo Day 9 suppl. It may get worse again, but today was better.

It was a delight to watch church at TBC on Facebook Live. Thank you tech team. It was good of Alex to substitute in the pulpit where I was to be substituting for Justin. And Ross, nothing says robust, healthy evangelical church like having a crusty retired US Army aviator read the scripture and lead in prayer.

Unaccountably, the owie on my tongue has hardly protested at all today, making chewing and swallowing much easier. I still do not have an appetite, but the prospect of serious pain when swallowing makes one look askance at yet another beef tip. So I ate tonight... like a reluctant 10 yr old, but I did eat.

Nurse says white bloods are at 0.2 and even that minimal level can repair some damage to the mouth sores. She is probably right, but you won't convince me those angels garbed as housekeepers last night was just coincidence.

But there still persists a low fever which makes lots of things tedious and unhappy.

Now that I know a little more about this malady I can say that I could have seen it at least 2 weeks earlier; Unusual purple and persistent bruising on extremities (low platelets); shortness of breath, sudden fatigue (low red blood cells); persistent swelling (low white blood cells). When those stars align, it's Leukemia, and when it comes on fast, it's Acute. Tests must prove it, but that's why the Andover Med Center people went to immediate Leukemia treatment mode.

A shout out to Clark S___ for coming up with a photo that's got to be 40 years old. Cool holiday sweater, huh!

I'll watch a little YouTube Peter Zeihan (thanks John L___) and then wait for the next oxycodone. Well, the day wasn't THAT good. Curt

July 07

Chemo Day 13 suppl. Spent a brief amount of time on a laptop this morning, mostly insurance related, and found it exhausting after about 10 minutes.

The Mobility Aide walked me a half mile twice today and explained that Floor 7 is a series of H-Shaped hallways that occasionally interconnect, meaning there are many box canyons requiring reverse direction. I explained to her that Stonewall Jackson faced the same issue in the Shenandoah Valley campaign in 1862, but used the succession of advance and retreat to confuse Union troops and give him some serious victories.

I am sure she internalized it, although I noted the big smile of relief when she deposited me back at my room.

Psalm 34:17 The righteous cry, and the LORD heareth, and delivereth them out of all their troubles. C

July 10

Chemo Day 16. The migraine pill did the trick and pushed the headache away almost entirely. Like any good 12 hour pill, it's effective for about 11 1/2 hours, then takes a half hour to ramp up, but it's much gooder today.

Lynn walked me a half mile this morning and because it's Sunday I wore the bright red Chemo kilt.

Have been battling a low grade fever for a week; the CT scan this morning showed little nodules of something in the lungs. Not pneumonia, but probably an airborne fungus. Or maybe an alien incursion of some kind... the doctor was wearing a mask and it was hard to hear exactly what she said. Anyway it gets treated with some goop from the juice bar, which might give me chills or not and might cause discomfort or not.

Yeah... whatever. Bring it on.

I think this one was from Kelly S___, good passage:

Chapter 7

Psalm 73:26 My flesh and my heart faileth: but God is the strength of my heart, and my portion for ever.

Enjoy your Sunday, with chills or not, and with discomfort or not! C

July 10

Chemo Day 16 suppl. I see that someone (Phill R___) ratted me out to the ATT/SBC crew so that many have reached out with good wishes and prayers. Very glad to hear from each of you! My world is mostly a 12x14 room and this CB site lets me at least look over the wall.

So we did the new anti fungus routine to kill lung nodules. It looks impressive, with 3 different bags of fluid slithering into my PIC lines at once. But as far as I can tell, it's a non-event. Not seeing any side effects yet.

Proverbs 25:25 As cold waters to a thirsty soul, so is good news from a far country.

One hour later: Not so fast, Red Leader. "Chills" barely does justice to it. And I don't even want to *think* about cold water, from a far country or otherwise.

July 11

Chemo Day 17 suppl. The lungus fungus has spreadus a little with a few red spots on back, scalp, chest, legs. They biopsied a couple today to see what's what, but we are already treating it with about every antibio available anyway.

And yeah, the chills returned tonight. Lynn and I, looking on the bright side, identified all the things that uncontrollable shrieking shaking chills are NOT: They are not nausea, diarrhea, migraine, abscess tooth, compound fracture at a remote mountain lake, federal indictment, IRS judgment. So enough whining already.

Reagan told of the 2 Russian workers who discussed the Soviet paradise. One said, Have we finally achieved it? The other replied, Oh [heck] no; it can get a lot worse than this.

Feasting on platelets and somebody else's blood tonight. Sleep well! C

July 12

Chemo Day 18 suppl. At least we are consistent; the lung fungus treatment acts the same way every day. Serious chills for about 2 hours and extreme fatigue. It is good to have predictability. This is day 3 of it and I don't have a guess on how long it will go.

A verse to use for that is the one that says, "there is no revelation from the Lord, we are in dire straits, and nobody knows how long this will last." (paraphrase). Just as well I can't find it because it's a real downer. Siri can't find it either.

So try this one instead:

Daniel 12:3 And they that be wise shall shine as the brightness of the firmament; and they that turn many to righteousness as the stars for ever and ever.

So go and ask God to turn someone to righteousness on your watch. Hang in there! Curt

July 14

Chemo Day 20. Actually, and this is a little embarrassing, there were NO chills after the lung fungus treatment last night. I was all ready: multiple blankets, warm blankets, tucked in all around… and a non-event. After 2 hours I threw off all the covers, moved down to a single sheet and a light blanket and slept the night through.

Staff: Well, that can happen, we suppose.

But I know better. Somebody is praying against the chills and exhaustion.

To channel James Cagney in Mister Roberts (1955): "Who did it? Who did it? You know who you are and I want to know who did it!"

We shall see if this happy condition persists.

John 15:7. If ye abide in me, and my words abide in you, ye shall ask what ye will, and it shall be done unto you.

Whoever is praying specifically against the chills, keep it up. I am ever grateful to you. Curt

~~~~~~~~~~~~~~~~~~~

Other Voices

I followed Curt's progress on Caring Bridge every day but did not post often. I struggled to find the right words most of the time.

When I saw his "to die for" statement about the protein shake [July 02], I couldn't resist. On the CB app, I commented: "Please avoid use of phrases such as 'to die for' during this time, even if in reference to such benign topics as protein shakes, unless they are quoted directly from the Bible. Thank you."

I wondered if he said that intentionally in reference to the near-death circumstances, or if it was just a turn of phrase used without any "pun-like" intentions. Either way, I decided to use it to try to make light of the situation; hopefully, my attempt at humor was at least understood if not actually funny.

I'm still curious to know, however, if that "to die for" statement was gallows humor or not. – Jeff

~~~~~~~~~~~~~~~~~~~

CB comment [July 02]: We've talked about this…no more gallows humor until this is over!!! – Lynn

~~~~~~~~~~~~~~~~~~~

Chapter 7

Inflection Point 2 – Catheter or not

I'm a big boy: 6 foot 4 inches, and when I checked in, I tipped the scales at 238 pounds. After four days of IV fluids, massive amounts of antibiotics and chemo drugs, I was at 281. I had gained 43 pounds virtually overnight.

It was all fluid, and unhappily most of it settled in my legs and feet, which swelled up like... well, like very fat legs and feet. I could not lift them to get out of bed without assistance.

Because of this, Doctor N returned with the next challenge.

He took his place in the chair facing me and explained the problem. "You have way too much fluid," he said. "This was to be expected, and it was important to get these antibiotics and chemo drugs started. But now," he paused, "we have a problem getting rid of it all."

"Why get rid of it?" I asked. "Won't it go away eventually?"

He shook his head. "The only way you lose the fluid is by excreting it. We have two ways of doing that. First," he said, "we could insert a catheter and let the bladder vacate as it will. That would be most comfortable for you. The other way is to let you urinate it out. The problem," he said, "is that with this much fluid, and with a diuretic to help, you will be standing at a toilet for 24 hours straight."

I was not exactly naive. I had been hospitalized before and knew that the experience of lying in a hospital bed with procedures performed by strangers violates every precious vestige of dignity. Most of life comes down to the visceral dimensions of what we might call inputs and outputs of the physical variety. Food and drink go in, and after specific internal organs have harvested their bounty, the leftovers must be removed.

Jesus pointed out (*Mark 7:18–19*) that what a man eats or drinks goes into the stomach and "out of the body." It was time for the first – but most certainly not the last – discussion of throughputs.

"Twenty-four hours," I observed. "That doesn't sound practical."

He shook his head. "Not only that," he said, "but it would overwhelm your kidneys, and you would most certainly suffer permanent kidney failure."

I pursed my lips. "That would mean... what? Dialysis?" It was something I knew virtually nothing about.

"Yes," he confirmed. "Kidney dialysis. Not a good solution."

"So, we do the catheter," I said. "That seems like an easy one."

He nodded slightly; then, his expression became more serious. "But we don't like that one either," he said, "because of the elevated risk. Your white blood cells are virtually non-existent, and platelets are also deficient."

I frowned. I knew that the bone marrow manufactured platelets, and it was not doing its job at present; but I had a question. "At the risk of admitting that I have forgotten everything I learned in 8th grade science class," I said, "what's a platelet?"

He smiled. "Platelets are what coalesce blood when you are injured. Without platelets, any cut or tear, virtually any damage that draws blood, regardless of how small, will continue to bleed."

"Until when?" I studied his expression and understood. "Until I bleed out," I guessed.

He nodded. "And here is the problem. Inserting the catheter always carries risk. It is a mechanical procedure, and there is a chance that it will snag the inside of the urethra at some point and cause bleeding. Normally this is not a concern, but normally we have platelets at work."

I began to see the problem but still had a question. "And how will we know if that has happened?" I asked.

He confidently replied, "There will be blood at the point of insertion."

"And then...?" I began.

His gaze steadied on me. "And then," he said slowly, "we will do for you what we can."

Chapter 7

I stared at him and wondered if these dramatic interludes would become a habit. It reminded me of Walt Whitman's *When Lilacs Last in the Door-Yard Bloomed*: "*I had the knowledge of death on one side of me, and the thought of death close by on the other.*" Not that I've read much of Walt Whitman. In fact, I think that's the only poem of his I've ever read.

I broke the silence. "So, if we can't catheterize, or urinate, is there another option?" But I already knew the answer.

"No," he asserted. "Furthermore," he added, "we must begin to remove that excess fluid immediately. The kidney damage will begin any time, and perhaps it already has. So here is what we will do."

I was getting used to this doctor. The quickening of his eye and the slight excitement in his voice told me he loved balancing risks and probabilities to produce successful outcomes. I concluded he was prone to aggressive action, but I supposed that was required in his line of business. Slow and steady would win no races against an aggressive cancer.

Despite the drama – and the stakes – I found myself loving it.

"We are going to use the catheter," he confirmed. "But first, we will give you a maximum number of platelets by IV. The most we can provide is 30,000. We are going to drip those into your system. Your body will not accept that quantity," he continued, "and many will begin to die within minutes of insertion." He smiled somewhat wickedly. "But some will survive," he said, "and the hope is that if there is a problem with the catheter, you may have just enough to stop the bleeding."

"So, you will drip the platelets," I said, "and then… what? You will do some test to determine how many platelets survive?"

"No," he said. "There will not be time, and there is no good way to take that measure short of a blood test. There is no point anyway. We will administer the platelets and then immediately insert the catheter." He paused. "And we will know soon enough if it works."

I nodded, musing that we would also know soon enough if it did *not* work. *We will do for you what we can*, ran through my mind. I realized that probably meant a morphine drip sufficient to ease one's passing. *Eegads*. At least Medicare was probably good for it.

"Well then, when do we start?"

He relaxed, and again, I caught the quickening of his eye. "Right away," he said with a note of boyish enthusiasm. "I have already ordered the platelets."

*****

The charge nurse in the cancer ward was a tough-as-nails twenty-something who could not be rattled by anything. She was pleasant, personable, flippant, happy-go-lucky, and enormously competent. She had no doubt done hundreds of catheter insertions in her young career. While she probably understood the risks better than the doctor, she was businesslike and put on an air of confidence. Maybe it was just for show, but it was a good show, and I was in no position to complain.

The platelet drip finished its course. She disconnected the tube to my PICC line and looked at me. "Okay, are you ready, Curt?" she asked.

"Bring it on," I said. "Take your best shot." I don't know that I felt confident, but I was determined not to show weakness.

She had everything ready and got right to work. The actual insertion took maybe ten seconds... and was wide-eyed excruciating. "Aarrgh!" I gasped. "What have you done!" I writhed in pain. "Honey, I've gotta say, you have done me dirty! What we had, you and I may never recover from this!"

She took the quasi-flirtation in stride. "But Sweetie," she protested, "I am only doing for you what you needed to be done. Just consider it one of those bumps in the road that every relationship experiences."

It became a private joke that we had this boy-girl thing going. Illogically, the catheter experience cemented our relationship, and we became good friends.

There was no blood at the point of insertion. It worked.

Let me back up a couple of days and explain the chemotherapy routine. A delightfully competent chemo nurse told Lynn and me what the process would look like. This first round of chemo was called Induction. It would last seven days and use a "7/3" approach: Seven days of a drip called Cytarabine, concurrent with three days of Idarubicin. Idarubicin (administered on days one through three) is highly aggressive in attacking and killing white blood cells. Cytarabine is more tame but still deadly to the whites.

A month after the Induction phase, and assuming it is successful in killing off the white blood cells, the patient customarily enters the Consolidation phase, which is ongoing chemotherapy. This is usually done a week at a time, one week out of four, and lasts through four cycles. Mine would ultimately go for six cycles rather than four, but that's for a later chapter. Let's try to survive Induction first.

The administration of the chemo drug resembles a process from a nuclear test facility. In the first place, two nurses must confirm the drug's administration. One reads aloud my name, date of birth and I.D. number from my bracelet; the other verifies my identity and makes a computer entry. I was reminded of the Minute Man silos from the 1970s where two operators were required to turn keys simultaneously to launch the nuke.

The administering nurse dresses in a full-coverage plastic suit and uses an oversize hypodermic affair (a clear cylinder an inch in diameter and about six inches long) to push the drug into my PICC line. The slurry itself is bright red, and the hypodermic resembles nothing so much as a grease gun. One of the CB followers said it reminded him of the red lithium grease he used on the ball joints in his '66 Chevy. He had a point.

While the nurse inserts the drug, using a plunger on the back of the cylinder, she watches the PICC attachments to ensure flow-through. She explained that there are four inspection points where she can visually confirm that the drug is being successfully inserted.

The process takes about half an hour. With some trepidation, I wondered what violence was being done to my white blood cells. On the other hand, the mutant whites, not too different from Jean-Luc Picard's Cyborgs, had turned on me and were in need of a good killing; I recalled hearing once that the point of chemotherapy is to kill the cancer before you kill the host. The race was on.

*****

I should point out the first of a few events that I can only see as miraculous. Unlike some, I am not given to reading miracles into unusual developments. My Christian experience has leaned toward the empirical rather than the supernatural. Nevertheless, I recognize that the Holy Spirit works even today in wondrous ways, and the power of prayer cannot be dismissed. If I needed proof of that, it first came in the person of Marva.

July 2 On the second Saturday of my confinement, a tall, black, cheerful, and robust female entered my room wearing the customary dark blue scrubs that identified her as a housekeeper. "My name is Marva," she declared, "and I'm to clean this room for a Mr. Curt." She took in the room with a housekeeper's practiced eye and settled on the exhausted-looking fellow in the bed. "Are you Mr. Curt?" she demanded. This dynamic woman sucked up all the oxygen in the room.

"That would be me," I managed to say. But my speech was slurred.

Chapter 7

Some history: As you would know, when I first determined I needed to see a urologist, I could not merely call for an appointment; back in May, I had first to see my PCP to ask "Mother, may I?" and get the referral. These are insurance rules over which we, in the proletariat, have no sway. At that initial visit, the PCP prescribed a water pill to help reduce swelling from my original complaint. After taking it for three days, black spots half the size of dimes began to appear inside my mouth. A few were on my tongue; they seemed to move to the inside cheek wall the next day. Mouth sores: They were an irritant but not overly so.

When they got worse over the next two days, it finally occurred to me that they were perhaps a side effect of the water pill, so I stopped taking it. The mouth sores continued. A blemish developed on the right side of my tongue, halfway back, that was becoming painful. The black spots continued to appear, first here, then there. Bizarre.

Hydrochlorothiazide, the water pill: I looked up that drug on the Mayo Clinic website and discovered scores of potential side effects listed. Among them were diarrhea, shortness of breath, fatigue, mouth sores, and muscle aches. *Ahh,* I thought, *mystery solved.*

But the mouth sore did not recede when I quit taking the pill. It later occurred to me to look up other drugs and their side effects. As a layman, I was chagrined to learn that virtually every drug in North America lists the same potential side effects: Diarrhea, shortness of breath, fatigue, mouth sores, and muscle aches. It's probably a liability thing; good thing the lawyers are watching out for me. So much for my amateur doctoring.

Mouth sores are often associated with various cancers. After discussing it with the oncologist and others, I concluded that this development was related to leukemia, not the water pill. But, *Oh, boy,* I had mouth sores to look forward to along with everything else.

Mouth sores are a needless distraction. They have absolutely nothing to do with surviving cancer. They serve only to make regular and necessary activities like speaking and swallowing painful. As though I have nothing else to deal with, lying on an uncomfortable bed in an institutional room, contemplating the end of my life, mouth sores are just plain mean.

By the time Marva showed up, I could barely swallow. It was vital for me to eat, of course, so the nurse and I had worked out a plan: Two hours before a meal, she administered Oxycodone; an hour before the meal, she administered Tylenol; and just before eating, I swabbed the inside of the mouth with Lidocaine to deaden everything. With the Oxycodone and Tylenol at peak efficiency and the tongue numbed, I could choke down some of my dinner. It was still painful. And just as bad, it affected my speech.

Some have said the only thing I do well is talk – where they get that notion, I have absolutely no idea. Having that capability compromised was disorienting.

Oxycodone produced other effects that were awe-inspiring, entertaining, and scary. One day, Lynn and her brother Ross sat on the couch facing me; the three of us were talking. Suddenly I noticed a tall, sandy-haired man clad in cargo pants and a yellow windbreaker standing near the door, only a few feet from the sofa.

I glanced at Lynn and Ross, then back to the door… nothing. He was gone. I rejoined the conversation, slightly wide-eyed, and said nothing about the visitor.

On another occasion, I found myself awake at 3:00 a.m. desperately searching the bedclothes for the cap to the tube of Chapstick. Coming fully awake, I checked the time, realized what I was doing, and sternly told myself, "There is no lid to the Chapstick! Go to sleep!"

"Fine!" I snapped at myself. Then I frantically began to beat the covers again, searching for the non-existent cap.

Oxycodone is a marvelous pill that produces wondrous experiences while it kills the pain. I desperately wanted to avoid it.

Marva picked up on my mood. "Mr. Curt, what you lookin' so down for? Don't you know this is the day the Lord hath made?"

As best I could, I explained the mouth sore and the extreme discomfort.

Marva leaped into action. It was as though she had been waiting for her chance. "Mr. Curt," she proclaimed in her booming voice, "Jesus do not want you sufferin' from mouth sores! We gonna pray against them mouth sores right now!"

And she did. Laying her hands on me, she closed her eyes and raised her face to the ceiling; when she began to speak to the Lord, it was clear she was on her home turf. This was no genteel and meek, "Oh dear Lord; we just thank you for this man…." No, Marva stormed the gates of Heaven and took Lynn and me along for the ride.

Delivered with great energy, it was something like, "Oh dear Jesus, You are high and lifted up, and Master of all this creation, and You are the most high and exalted Lord! You are the Creator and the Lord of this man's mouth! You made this man's mouth, and You can fix this man's mouth! We ask You right now to rebuke that mouth sore that afflicts Mr. Curt. Right now, Lord! Heal his mouth and his tongue so that he may be able to eat and swallow and speak without pain! Banish the devil who cometh only to steal and kill and destroy, and give peace and healing and comfort to Mr. Curt so that he may praise you freely and testify to your incredible saving grace!" And so on and on. This lasted for maybe five minutes.

Afterward, I was physically and spiritually drained.

Through unaccustomed tears, I clutched Marva's hand in both of mine and tried to thank her, but the emotions overflowed, and I could not squeak out more than a feeble "Thank you!" This is a little embarrassing for a tough guy like me… but it was the first of many events where the buttons got pushed, and I choked up.

Marva mopped the floor, took out the trash, and left, promising to return later to look in on me.

July 4 But here's the thing: By the following day, I kid you not, there was no more mouth sore. I could still feel it on the side of my tongue, but there was no discomfort and only minor pain. Soon, we stopped Oxycodone. For the next three months, there was not a single recurrence of mouth sore. The blemish disappeared in about a week, and I could not tell where it had been. Miracle? Yes. There is no denying it, and that's what I'm going with.

Lynn and I watched our church service Sunday morning on the Facebook Live broadcast, but we had already had worship that weekend.

I asked a doctor the next day for a clinical explanation of the reduction of the mouth sore. He explained that something like that is only healed by native white blood cells attacking it. He said antibiotics would not fix that problem; they could only perhaps prevent the onset of such a problem. I pointed out that I had virtually no white blood cells operating.

"Yes, I know," he said and shrugged. "But everyone is different; many people suffer from mouth sores due to leukemia, but others don't."

"But I did suffer from a mouth sore," I insisted. "I've had it for a week or more. And suddenly, this morning, it's gone."

He shrugged again. "Can't explain it," he said, "but we all react differently to various drugs and antibiotics."

I don't fault him for his answer. I probably would have said the same to a patient in that situation.

A chaplain friend of mine, Rob, later told me that physicians frequently use the term "spontaneous remission" to explain unexpected developments like this. It allows them to admit the reality of miraculous healings without taking sides in a spiritual debate. This made sense to me; I appreciate that many doctors have solid Christian principles, which probably influenced many of them to take that career. Others don't. Whatever the orientation, I applaud the professionalism and clinical competence.

As a post-script to this, Marva came by a few days later. I told her the happy result of her prayer, and she did not seem at all surprised. I said, "I'm glad you came back, though, because I want to check your St. Francis I.D. Are you a real employee, or are you an angel?"

She laughed and showed me her card. "I'm just a housekeeper," she said. "This is the ministry God has called me to!" Embarrassingly, I cried again. Sheesh, what a wuss.

July 10 I had noted for a few days that when my vitals were taken, the nurse indicated I was running a slight fever, maybe one degree.

What's one degree of fever to a macho man like me?

But Doctor A took it seriously. "You have an infection," she declared. "Otherwise, you would not be running this fever. I have ordered a CT scan to see what's going on."

Mayo Clinic: *A computerized tomography (CT) scan combines a series of X-ray images taken from different angles around your body and uses computer processing to create cross-sectional images (slices) of the bones, blood vessels and soft tissues inside your body. CT scan images provide more detailed information than plain X-rays do.*

Sure... I knew all that. It's like an X-ray on steroids. The CT scan is distinct from the MRI. Before we were done, I would see both. But, for the patient who may tend to claustrophobia, the CT is a happier experience than the MRI.

The Mayo, again: *Magnetic resonance imaging (MRI) is a medical imaging technique that uses a magnetic field and computer-generated radio waves to create detailed images of the organs and tissues in your body.*

In the CT lab, I lay on a table that slid me inside a cylindrical contraption, reminding me of a torture machine from an old *Man from U.N.C.L.E.* episode. I was instructed to raise my arms above my head, bending at the elbows and stretching them backward unnaturally and uncomfortably. The idea was to avoid obstructing the view of the chest with my arms, and not to let them touch the roof of this small cave inches from my face.

The round Hobbit-door-like opening of the machine was barely large enough to accommodate my considerable carcass; it was uncomfortable but not intolerable. A mechanized voice was imperious: "Hold your breath!" An LED light counted down from an illumined "6". Reaching "1," the voice commanded, "Breathe!"

A flywheel spun somewhere, and a small aperture in the curved surface just above my face showed that a large cylinder encompassing my entire body and the bed was spinning around me.

I supposed I could have invented that machine, given enough time. Or not.

The bed slid forward and back, bumping my elbows against the low ceiling. Then, with me holding my breath and releasing it on command of The Voice, the process was repeated three or four times as the bed was pushed various distances into the bowels of this spinning dynamo. I took this to mean the actual lens, or whatever you might call it, had to be positioned over the section of the body in question.

It was over in four or five minutes, and I was returned to my room.

The following day, Doctor A came back. "You have half a dozen tiny nodules on your lungs," she said. "I don't think they are pneumonia, which might be expected, but they don't look like pneumonia. We are not sure what they are, but we suspect a fungus of some type."

I nodded. "More drugs?" I asked.

"More drugs," she affirmed. "We will use an all-purpose fungus treatment until we figure out what this is."

So? I thought. Just more IV activity. It was an issue for the nurses but not for me… until that afternoon.

Lynn caught a nurse. "Look at his back, would you please?" she asked. "There are two new red spots on the shoulders that we have not seen before." She gestured to the blemishes, and the nurse frowned. "We'll have the doctor look at them," she said. "They look maybe like a fungus."

Ah-hah… *Fungus this, fungus that,* I thought. *Just throw some drugs at it.*

But they were already throwing drugs at it, and here we had a couple of new spots – a half dozen on the lungs and two on the back.

July 11 By the time a doctor looked at it two hours later, there were more: Scalp, legs, hands. This fellow moved fast. The following day, with over two dozen spots, half an inch in diameter, across my body, they took a punch biopsy of the two on my back.

A punch biopsy is the size of a paper punch. They position some mechanism above the spot (it was on my back, so I could not see it) and stab the subject location with a small round tool that collects a sample of the skin. A technician explained that it would take the infected area, along with some natural skin next to it, in a divot the size of a paper punch. I imagined it to be like a Venn diagram.

Off it went to the Mayo Clinic, and the most significant impact on me was trying not to scratch my scalp where the infections were. The other, more minor but frustrating effect was that one site was between two toes on my left foot.

A sore had formed in the V between toes two and three, down in the wedge between the piggies where it could not be seen or touched and where air would never reach it. It would take weeks to heal.

I was becoming short-tempered with the fungus. *This is just not fair. Come out in the open where I can see you!*

And it got worse: Mayo replied with the identity of this fungus. It was called Fusarium, and it was bloodborne. That meant it was not spread by physical contact like any self-respecting athlete's foot. Instead, it reaches the circulatory system and could appear anywhere on or in the body. Anyplace, any organ. Like the Holy Ghost, it *goeth whither it willeth (John 3:8 – sort of – KJV).*

That sounded quite ominous. And it was, but the treatments proceeded.

*****

During the chemotherapy treatment, other drugs are administered, some by drip and some by pill. One of the standard drugs is amphotericin; it is not used often, and I will not hazard to say why it's used for some patients and not others. It is an antibiotic to guard against fungus infection. The staff calls it "ampho-terrible," and for good reason.

A doctor (one of the three dozen, I have no idea which) explained that in *some* cases, *some* patients report *some* mild chills that *might* occur an hour after the drip is completed. I have learned that when doctors qualify statements of side effects in this manner, running and hiding might be a good idea.

The first night I received amphotericin during the Induction phase, I laid in bed for an hour after the drip finished and convinced myself it wasn't so bad. I had no side effects; *I must be the tough guy I have been telling everyone I am.*

And then the wind came up.

Discounting the reality that I was in a secure room in a brick-and-mortar building in the middle of Kansas, a sudden gust of cold air from the Arctic north suddenly swept my bed. Although the room remained silent, it seemed to shriek like a banshee and seized me with chills I did not know were possible.

I shook, I chattered, I trembled violently. I could hardly hold my hand steady to push the "Help me, I've fallen and can't get up" button on the nurse's remote. The bed shook. The impression of windows rattling and books falling off the table was strong.

Okay, it was merely a chill. But why understate the drama? It was unbelievably cold. No wonder they called this ampho-terrible. Nurses brought me warm blankets; not enough, but as futile gestures go, it was a nice effort.

I shook for over two hours, and then the fever broke, the chills receded, and left me a shivering, gasping wreck. Tough guy, right? The sheets were drenched with sweat. *In some cases, some patients report some mild chills that might set in.*

Chapter 7

July 13 This happened three nights in a row, and I spent each of the following days dreading the subsequent onset. How long could this go on?

I had put this on Caring Bridge, of course... why not let my constituency share the pain? And somebody started praying. I know this – I am convinced – because after the third night and after my detailed CB descriptions, there were suddenly no more chills.

Say what? There were no more chills? Not any.

I was ready with extra blankets, nurses on call to bring warm blankets on a moment's notice... I had done everything except pray, which was precisely the wrong direction. But somebody in the CB posse – I have no idea who – recognized what was required and acted. They prayed, and God answered. There is no other explanation.

Like the mouth sores, I asked a doctor for a clinical explanation the next day. "Some people have chills, and some don't," he said. "Can't explain it." The amphotericin treatment continued for the prescribed two weeks, and the chills never returned.

I learned something important about the church's role in bearing one another's burdens. This was real life, and honest prayer is part of the package.

Theological Contemplations

Doctor N was a man of action. Over the summer months, I concluded he did not know much about insurance, but he was all over cancer. The quickness of his eye and the enthusiasm with which he explained options – all of them poor, usually – belied a passion for healing that could not be hidden.

I had the distinct impression he was in a strategy game with life-and-death consequences and was playing to run up the score. He would have been at home with chess, 19th-century infantry combat, high technology salesmanship, or calling football plays; the strategy was the thing, and he loved to win. He was good at it.

Not a bad man to have on your side, weighing risks and estimating probabilities when your own life is on the line. He put me in mind of King David, who wrote, *With your help I can advance against a troop; with my God I can scale a wall (Psalm 18:29)*. Such unbridled, unapologetic optimism.

I could also not avoid the comparison with Joshua, who saw the angel with a drawn sword and challenged him: *Are you for us or for our enemies? (Joshua 5:13)*. About every other time in Scripture, when an angel appeared to a person, the first thing out of the angel's mouth was, "Do not be afraid." Clearly, the human was in fear. Probably Joshua was, too, but it did not stop him from meeting the threat head-on.

I loved it. As Tim Conway frequently commented to Ernest Borgnine: "Gee, I love that kind of talk!" *(McHale's Navy, ABC-TV, 1962)*

Interestingly, this attitude was not confined to the doctor staff. The charge nurse with the catheter assignment evidenced much the same determination. Cancer is a killer, and there are rarely good options for treatment. When the doctor ordered one, she took it and the risks in stride: *This we shall do*. Never let 'em see you sweat.

Once I got some distance from Whitman's *knowledge of death on one side of me and the thought of death close by on the other,* I reflected on the incredible maturity of a 27-year-old woman to accept such responsibility with steady hands. My respect for her shot up immeasurably.

Chapter 7

A clear-eyed assessment of the situation coupled with determined execution may not always work... but if success is ever to be had, this will always be required. Somehow, I had intuited this when I first showed up in the cancer ward, hence my "tough guy" persona. I wonder if this comes naturally to others. It did not come naturally to me as a pre-teen. Still, somewhere between then and now – starting with Tubby the Tuba and a comparative-advantage debate strategy – it took root in me.

~~~~~~~~~~~~~~~~~~~~

Other Voices

When I heard that Curt was seriously ill, my first thought turned out to be my default thought about him. That is, I have had the privilege of seeing the fruits of his faithfulness and witness play out on a daily basis for the last 33.5 years. He and Lynn helped set the stage for my wife, Amy, to become the powerful woman of God that she is today. Curt is and will always be an unparalleled model as a father, husband, employee, scholar... and Christmas Letter author. – Bill

~~~~~~~~~~~~~~~~~~~~

When I was discharged from the hospital, I received an email from a friend, a woman whom I had counseled a few times when she was going through a divorce. I was honored to be her go-to spiritual advisor. A lab report had shown a tumor; she was distraught. "I have read your CB posts," she said, "and I'm just not brave like you are. I don't do well with pain and am really afraid."

So... how do you answer *that*? "Suck it up, lady!" seemed a little uncaring and rude.

Eventually, I shared with her Psalm 118:5, my standby passage in times of stress and uncertainty: *When hard pressed, I cried to the Lord; he brought me into a spacious place.* King James Version: *...a wide place.* I don't know if that satisfied her, but the biopsy returned negative, and the problem seemed to disappear for the moment.

It still left me feeling inadequate to offer any absolute comfort. But to be fair, what is one *supposed* to say? Anything we come up with will either be insufficient or condescending, without much daylight between them.

In one of our small adult groups at church a few years ago, we tackled the subject head-on: How to help those in the throes of sudden disaster? Through discussion and shared frustration, we finally developed a job aid called "Ministering Through Tragedy." We printed it on three-inch square cards intended to be tucked into a Bible and forgotten until needed.

It sported a few Bible verses (Habakkuk 3:19 *The Sovereign Lord is my strength*; Romans 12:15 *Mourn with those who mourn*) and identified the Four P's of ministry, self-explanatory:

Practical – Casserole, childcare, housekeeping, lawn care.

Present – Be physically present and perhaps silent.

Pray – Offer a very brief prayer for them.

Peripheral – Be aware of others affected in the background.

Part of our discussion was whether to reduce such a challenging and profound task to mere alliterative talking points. I halfway apologized to the class: "Sorry to minimize such a deep issue by making it a trite acronym." However, Allison, an efficient and very busy mother of four, immediately opined: "Oh no, I'll take the acronym, please. Anything to make it easy to remember." And it stuck.

A few years earlier, during my tech career, I had been assigned a clerk, a charming and competent lady some ten years my senior. She came to work one morning a little less than her usual chipper self; she avoided eye contact and did her duties without speaking.

In a few minutes, she entered my office to arrange some reports and file papers. I asked her, "Are you all right today? You look a little down."

She turned to look at me, and the dam burst. Through sudden tears, she related that a teenage niece had been killed in a car wreck the previous night in Missouri.

I was on my feet, and in violation of everything holy in the employee handbook, I embraced her and let her cry. I was able to mutter in her ear, "He heals the brokenhearted and binds up their wounds," and said a brief prayer for her and the family.

It was wholly inadequate for the situation, but I reiterate: What is one *supposed* to say?

If we believe that the Word of God has the power to heal, strengthen and redeem, then it should be put to the test. Paul says the Gospel is the power of God for salvation (Romans 1:16); and if that is true, then we should probably just let it do its thing. I have concluded that God can use any piece of Scripture we share to accomplish His will, and it doesn't make much difference whether it is on-topic or not.

Once upon a time, I was at a church work camp in Kentucky. For about 20 years, Fred and I, from our local church, along with Louis and Alene from a neighboring community, had taken a group of about two dozen adults and high schoolers to Redbird Mission, a United Methodist Conference in southeast Kentucky, to help with local work projects: Roof repair, home remodeling, plumbing and electrical, about anything that needed doing in an economically very depressed community.

The point, of course, was to engage the teens in Bible study and "spiritual journey" discussions throughout the week. Alene issued a challenge in a large group meeting on the first night of this trip. "On Friday night, our last night together here, I want each of you to share your favorite Bible verse with the group."

One of the boys, whom I called Wildman, came to me that night in a near panic. "Curt!" he cried. "What's my favorite verse? What am I supposed to say?"

He had not brought his Bible along, of course... why would I expect him to bring his Bible along to church camp, anyway? So, I loaned him a Bible, gave him a 3x5 card and a pen, and asked him to copy 1 Peter 5:8. *Be alert and of sober mind. Your enemy the devil prowls around like a roaring lion looking for someone to devour.*

He said, "Oh yeah! Cool verse!" as he contemplated the word picture of the salivating predator stalking prey in the Savannah.

On the roofing crew that week, I challenged him. "Wildman! Who's your enemy?"

"The devil!"

"Who's he looking for?"

"Someone to devour!"

By Thursday night, he had the short verse memorized word-perfect, with reference, and approached me after supper. "Curt," he said, quieter than usual. "What do you think that verse means?"

I studied him. "Maybe lots of things. What do *you* think it means?"

He stared at the ground, avoiding my eyes. "I think it means the devil wants to eat me up."

I let his response hang in the air, and the atmosphere was suddenly charged. "Do you think that's right?" I asked.

No eye contact. He gulped. "Well... yes."

After some discussion, he prayed to ask God to forgive his sins; he asked Jesus to enter his heart and make him a new creation. At the following night's meeting, he shared his favorite verse, 1 Peter 5:8. He quoted it with vigor and confidence, to the delight and dismay of peers and adults.

If the Word has power, then it has power. Our role is to let it work.

Chapter 7

Through the Caring Bridge journaling, I also learned some things about the church's role. The amphotericin was truly ampho-terrible. While I didn't think it would kill me, the prospect of the nightly chills was unbearably discouraging. It compromised my self-appointed role as the tough guy. Fear entered my 12x14 room and crouched in the corner, watching and waiting, salivating like that lion in the tall grass. *This will never do,* I thought.

Nobody knew it then, but by July 10th, I was less than three weeks into an 83-day ordeal. That was the first night of amphotericin. The following day, I put it on Caring Bridge, explaining the misery, and repeated the narrative for the next three days. I was careful to keep my tone upbeat (perhaps a little snarky), but my message was clear: This is a terrible situation and needs intervention.

And then deliverance. On July 14, I wrote: *...there were NO chills after the lung fungus treatment last night. I was all ready: multiple blankets, warm blankets, tucked in all around... and a non-event. Finally, after two hours, I threw off all the covers, moved down to a single sheet and a light blanket and slept the night through.*

Somebody had prayed, and that was that. Galatians 6:2 *Carry each other's burdens, and in this way you will fulfill the law of Christ.*

I'm still not sure I know what "the law of Christ" is, but I learned of the symbiotic relationship we share in the Church. In this context, my role was to share the need; the Church's role was to carry that burden. In this case, they couldn't bear the burden by mowing my lawn or fixing my roof, but only by praying against the ampho-terrible. They did so admirably, and no one ever admitted to it.

Sharing the need, however, was uncomfortable. I would far rather be the strong one above pain and fear, an object of admiration and respect... and all that other irrelevant hooey. But that's not the way it works. Sometimes we just flat need help, and the sooner we admit it, the better.

The outcome would not have been good if either the church or I had abdicated our Scriptural responsibility. Okay... so deliverance probably would have arisen from another quarter (Esther 4:14), but both the church and I would have missed the blessing of obedience. It never works out well to refuse the leading of God.

It has led me to conclude: Don't suffer in silence... and also don't suffer in public.

A woman Lynn and I know was diagnosed with cancer about ten years ago. While we were not close to the family, we were aware of the diagnosis.

She dropped off my radar. We noted that she had disappeared from various venues where we had been accustomed to seeing her, but we knew nothing of her situation and did not have a convenient way to find her status. I had other priorities at the time, and because she was not in my orbit of close friends, I did not try to chase down information on her.

During my cancer event, she reached out to communicate with me. She has been battling cancer for many years, and like most of us, there are good and bad days. Her interest, along with everyone else's comments, incentivized me to stay in the fight. It would have been encouraging to have followed her progress, or lack thereof, over the last decade.

But how was I to know? Don't get me wrong: I don't want to hear a complete recitation of disillusionment and despair, but being informed at a 10,000-foot level would facilitate prayer and encouragement. My experience with the Big C is that if you lose the attitude war, you lose the war.

This, therefore, is my appeal: When you face a serious threat to yourself, or your other, or your child, please: *Don't suffer in silence... and also don't suffer in public.* Let us know what goes on so that we may be the Church.

Chapter 7

Okinawa, 1945

Dick Atkins, a Texas boy, was 14 years old on a December Sunday morning when Japanese forces surprised-attacked the U.S. naval base at Pearl Harbor.

Filled with a teenager's impatient visions of glory, he was anxious to join up. On his seventeenth birthday, his parents agreed to sign the release, allowing him to join the Navy. His biggest worry was that the war would be over before he could get into it. He told the recruiter he wanted the job that had the shortest training stream, and in a highly unusual twist, he got what he asked for. He was assigned to an LCVP (Landing Craft Vehicle Personnel) unit.

Young Dick was the "Captain" of a Chris-Craft boat that held 36 Marines, supervising three other sailors under his command. His crew supported the invasion of Okinawa, truly the last Marine beachhead of World War II. He had made it, but just barely.

As his boat idled in the mother ship's flooded cargo bay, waiting to swim out and load Marines, the propeller became tangled in a piece of floating rope. His LCVP was immediately latched onto by an overhead hoist and winched upward out of the way, so as not to impede the departure of those behind him.

Atkin's boat had been written off. He had enlisted, been trained, and sailed 10,000 miles to be sidelined at the last possible moment.

With incredible courage, only available to the young, inexperienced, and bullet-proof, he hung suspended 30 feet above the roiling water, his feet propped on the nearby catwalk while one of his sailors held him.

He could barely reach the screw with the tip of his combat knife, and tediously began to saw through the entangling saltwater-soaked line. He finished just in time to be lowered back into the disembarkation bay and join the last rank of the landing flotilla.

It didn't end there. They loaded the Marines, made the run to shore under only light small-arms opposing fire, and dropped the warfighters "feet dry" on the sandy beach. As Atkins backed away from the beach to return for a second load, he saw a half dozen Japanese soldiers come sprinting toward his boat and the boat adjacent to him. Because of the positions of the two LCVPs, neither could bring their gunwale-mounted machine guns to bear on the enemy group. Atkins and one of his sailors grabbed their personal M-1 carbines and opened fire on the advancing troops. They each emptied two magazines of .30 caliber round ball and stopped the threat.

He didn't start to shake until out in the open harbor, on his way back for the next load of Marines.

It was his very first action in the war... 17 years old. He had not thought there was even a remote chance he would ever need his carbine, but it stayed close by his side, locked and loaded, on every subsequent trip. (*American Sailor*, Anchor Publishing Company, 2006, p. 277.)

*****

Most of us will never land Marines on a beach under enemy fire. But understanding the critical roles of assessment and execution goes a long way toward slaying our dragons, whether emotional, financial, relational, spiritual... or canceral. (I just made that one up.)

One other tiny detail: Amphotericin, Idarubicin, Cytarabine, Oxycodone, Tylenol, and all those other foreign agents form something of a devil's brew inside a pure and pristine body such as my own.

These agents are not idle; I don't know their relationship to one another, but in my layman's imagination, they combine, mix, roil, and simmer. And then they think up mischief: How can we best remind Curtis that we are here and that, for some reason, we are not happy?

Chapter 8

Caring Bridge Journal, July 14 – July 19, 2022

July 14
Chemo Day 20 SPECIAL. The principal oncologist is back from vacation now, and announces that we are doing the bone marrow biopsy today, not tomorrow. I think this is because he can get results from the local lab by tomorrow and not have to wait till next week. This bone marrow biopsy is fairly important and could probably benefit from your prayer. C

July 14
Chemo Day 20 suppl. I am glad the CB interface cannot display the tears. I am absolutely overwhelmed by your love and prayers.

Ok, enough squishy… on to hard news.

Biopsy: Left hip, a few unpleasant twinges but basically a non event. Results tomorrow. Looking for <5% blasts (bad White Blood cells) which would indicate effective chemotherapy, and then start talking remission. >5% is a very different conversation.

Lung fungus: per Onc Doc, this could be caused by the leukemia but in this case it is not. IDK how he knows. It is uncomfortable but not debilitating. So, another 10 days antibiotics to fix that. This is the routine that causes the chills, or not. But no chills again tonight. Those chills are afraid of the prayers of the saints. Just as the mouth sores are. I do not speak in jest.

Headache: a 12 hour migraine seems to have fixed that.

Down for the night now. Maybe a shower tomorrow!

Exodus 17:12 But Moses' hands were heavy; and they took a stone, and put it under him, and he sat thereon; and Aaron and Hur stayed up his hands, the one on the one side, and the other on the other side; and his hands were steady until the going down of the sun.

Don't quit now! Curt

July 15
Chemo Day 21 RESULTS. Onc Doc: Good news. Not out of danger yet but bone marrow biopsy shows good results. More later. Curt.

Exodus 15:1. Then sang Moses and the children of Israel this song unto the LORD, and spake, saying, I will sing unto the LORD, for he hath triumphed gloriously: the horse and his rider hath he thrown into the sea.

July 16

Chemo Day 22 suppl. Mayo Clinic analyzed the lung fungus and St Francis has changed up the Ampho drip accordingly. Nobody knows how long but if we can keep other infections away, then in 3-4 days there might be enough homegrown WB cells they can get in the game.

Continue to pray the chills away; likewise the mouth sore. Prayer works, but to quote Han Solo, Don't get cocky.

Got a unit of blood today, which means the marrow production is not quite spooled up yet. But platelet levels are good, whether from an injection of them yesterday, or some minimal native production, that's good news.

We get twin injections daily of some goop that encourages WB production. They go into the belly. What I know about a gut shot I have learned from John Wayne and Clint Eastwood. Those sources now appear to be a little questionable. These are bare pinpricks, only surface deep.

Ephesians 6:12. For we wrestle not against flesh and blood, but against principalities, against powers, against the rulers of the darkness of this world, against spiritual wickedness in high places.

If we lose the attitude war, we lose the war. Hang tough! Curt

July 17

Chemo Day 23. At 900p last night in a routine check of vitals, BP was good, temp was normal, and pulse was 135. I objected, as my resting should be 56 or so. We have had lots of mechanical trouble with the pulse/ox finger stall gizmo this week. A flurry of activity, yes it really is 135, then calls to Onc Doc, Cardio Doc, portable EKG tech. Terms like Atrial Fibrillation and Arrhythmia crept into the conversation.

The upshot is they prepared a new cocktail drip to get the heart under control and wired me for remote monitoring with half a dozen adhesive pads to the chest.

I am told there is absolutely no interaction or interference with the Ampho treatment for the lung fungus. We are doing both simultaneously while also staying on the conventional antibiotics.

But we were up all night and a nurse's aide brought me a PBJ at 300am. Hah! An act of kindness!

And now here I am at 25 or 6 to 4, waiting for the break of day. (Chicago, 1970)

Late morning: no hemogoblins or platelets are required today, meaning the marrow is now contributing to the cause. Best of all, WB cell counts are up from 0.2 to 0.4. Onc Doc says once we see the levels begin to rise, they may shoot up pretty rapidly.

So, some very good news, but we are not out of it yet.

Chapter 8

I think maybe Steve B___ came up with this one:

Isaiah 8:13 Sanctify the LORD of hosts himself; and let him be your fear, and let him be your dread.

Enjoy your day of rest! Since I was up all night I plan to sleep lots today… in about 30 minute segments. Curt

July 18

Chemo Day 24 SPECIAL. Review: Leukemia is headed the right direction, lung fungus is being managed but may take some time, the heart arrhythmia remains pegged at about 140-160 pulse.

We have been on the arrhythmia drip for 3 days with no effect. A prolonged very fast rate = certain blood clots, so action is required.

Today we will do an electric shock to the heart hoping to find a Reset button.

Many risks attend this (one being stroke), but there has not been a major procedure yet without substantial risk.

Psalm 73:25-26 Whom have I in heaven but thee? and there is none upon earth that I desire beside thee. My flesh and my heart faileth: but God is the strength of my heart, and my portion for ever.

On a lighter note, Hilary had a Reset button that I don't believe was ever used. I wonder where that one got to? Curt

July 18

Lynn's status report, hospital stay day 27.

If you all could pray for something specific please. Curt's heart rate has been elevated for 3 days now and has not responded to the meds they have him on to reduce his heart rate. So they are going to shock his heart at 4:00 today. It should get the heart back in rhythm. But there are, as always, some negative things that could happen too. Even tho we had a good report Sunday, we are a long way from done. I personally count on knowing that this great cloud of witnesses is supporting me with love and prayer even tho I can't see you. I know you are there and working on my behalf. And Curt's also.

May all that happens here be done for the glory of God.

July 18

They're running late but the procedure is done. I'll post this brief message. The procedure was successful and his heart is back in rhythm. Thank you all for praying and to God be the glory. Lynn

July 18

Chemo Day 24 suppl.

Ok, so that seemed to work, thanks in no small part to your prayers. Cardio Doc zapped me once and somehow that made the atrium sit up and pay attention. Apparently in atrial fibrillation the aorta fires off many random electric commands. It is supposed to generate a single command in rhythm with the ventricle to accomplish the lub-dub routine. All those random impulses are not sustainable.

The electric shock to the heart is not preferred, but with all my other attendant conditions it was about the only option still in play. In the case, it was sort of a non-event. I think we have to assess for a couple of days to declare success but at this point the heart monitor tells me we are in the 80-90 pulse range.

Again, thanks for your prayers. I'll watch a little Dennis Prager U and then see if I can sleep. Curt

July 19

Chemo Day 25 (hospital day 28). Cardio Doc visited early today and I congratulated him on the successful shock treatment yesterday. He was beaming like a young boy, said it worked just like it's supposed to.

Imagine my delight and surprise when I received a text with a music video from Brian H___. He and Charlie S___ are the trumpet players in a pre-Covid brass quintet called Patina, along with a trombone, a French horn and me on tuba. I had been asked about favorite hymns or tunes but hadn't known why.

Those guys live recorded Savior Like a Shepherd Lead Us and America the Beautiful. I doubt you will find either of those pieces arranged purely for trumpet duet, which means Brian probably developed original arrangements himself.

Brian and Charlie both play well above my level (as do the other Patinas), and when I opened the text and saw what it was I cranked up the bluetooth and laughed and cried my way through both numbers several times. Guys, you have no idea how much that lifts my spirits.

On to medico: The arrhythmia seems to have been arrested, pulse is sort of normal at 75-90, still monitoring it. New WB cells are at 2.0 today, twice yesterday's level. RB cells and platelets are holding where they should be. The lung fungus (proper term Fusarium) seems to be in retreat but is devilishly difficult to exterminate, so prolly a few more days of that antibiotic drip.

Some swelling in lower extremities remains an issue.

Patiently waiting for the White Blood Cell army to build up; I think we want a count of 5.0.

Psalm 5:3 My voice shalt thou hear in the morning, O LORD; in the morning will I direct my prayer unto thee, and will look up.

Now please get back to work! Curt

Chapter 8

Inflection Point 3 – Your Heart is All A-flutter

July 15 With the 7/3 Cytarabine and Idarubicin Induction phase complete, it was time for the bone marrow biopsy. If one were looking for a Moment of Truth, this might rank right up there near the top.

The procedure meant they would bore a hole in the side of my rump with an auger, extract some of the soft and juicy bone marrow, feed it into a machine and let it sort out the contents. They were looking for the presence (or rather the absence) of "blasts," those immature genetically deviant FLT-3 (pronounced "flit three") white blood cells.

If the marrow contained less than five percent blasts, they could declare the chemo had worked, and the leukemia was – for now – in remission. Otherwise... well, they never told me what would have occurred otherwise. Perhaps another 7/3 round of chemo, or we would advance directly to a bone marrow transplant.

The biopsy itself produced nowhere near the discomfort I had expected. The prospect of a burly fellow turning a stainless-steel T-handle instrument (like the tap-and-die set I inherited from the farm) to invade deep into my hip was enough to challenge any tough guy. But as it turned out, the site was deadened so well that there was only a twinge or two when he reached the sweet spot.

Well and good... and then the wait for results.

There was sort of a lot hanging on those results.

We entertained grandkids. They were a little frustrated and perhaps intimidated by the hospital room and that they had to keep their distance from Grandpa, but they seemed to take it in stride. My CB journal entry from July 15: *I tried to explain to Corbin (g-son aged 8) that hospitals get all their blood from pirate battles bc we all know that pirates are always getting into sword fights. All their extra blood is collected in wooden barrels and shipped to various hospitals and kept in the basement. When some is needed they go down there and ladle out some into little plastic bags. He looked at me somewhat askance.*

Granddaughter Elizabeth (age 6) wanted to bring a flower or a potted plant for Grandpa; sweet of the little princess to think of me. But her mother explained that living plants are not allowed because of the potential presence of mold or fungus. Elizabeth, non-plussed but still pitching, asked, "So then, would a *picture* of a flower be okay?"

"I am sure it would," her mother replied, straight-faced. "If you draw a picture for Grandpa, that would be just as good."

So she did; it included flowers, grass, a few clouds, and a yellow sun with rays, which I was sure satisfied my minimum daily requirement for vitamin D. Lynn posted it to the wall of my room.

~~~~~~~~~~~~~~~~~~

Other Voices

Today, I get to do a hospital visit. Not have to... I get to. Why the enthusiasm, you ask? Because it's fascinating.... no, it's enlightening, to watch hospital staff enter a cancer patient's room with obvious smiles on their mask-covered faces. Now, I'm guessing they do this for all their patients, but in Curt's room, something about it is different. Almost like a God-ordained, two-way connection always takes place. And that is a gift to be able to see!
– Justin, Pastor

~~~~~~~~~~~~~~~~~~

After the family was gone, two nurses returned. It was not time for vitals or meds, making this an unusual visit. One came right to the point. "I cannot give you complete results of your biopsy," she said, "but I have seen the preliminary report. I wanted to tell you that your bone marrow is normal; no cancer is present; all is good."

I stared at her, wide-eyed, unspeaking. She continued. "The doctor will be in tomorrow to cover it with you, but we thought you should know as soon as we heard." She smiled. "So don't ask me any technical questions about it because I won't know the answers. But we wanted you to know."

I missed the last part of her short speech, overcome with sudden emotion. I had not realized until then the enormity of the stress I felt, wondering if this chemo gig had worked. The grandkids' visit, the pirate story, the flower picture, and the cancer readout did their work: I wept shamelessly and shook uncontrollably as she held my hand.

I am such a wuss.

*****

Drugs do funny things to people, even to tough guys. When there are lots of drugs, they can do seriously funny things. Sometimes they interact in particular ways that bring about entirely unrelated and unpredictable phenomena. Sometimes the phenom can be deadly.

July 16 On the heels of the biopsy, good news, I felt much better about my prospects for survival and almost missed the Next Big Thing. Getting ready for bed (surely a misnomer, as I had been in it nearly all day), a nurse took my vitals as usual. She intoned the results as she entered them into a computer terminal: "BP 115 over 65, pulse 135, temp 98.1, oxygen 94 percent."

"Wait," I said. "What's the pulse?"

"It says 135," she replied and pursed her lips. "That seems pretty high."

"It can't be that high," I replied. "Recheck it."

She did, and it was the same. "That's odd," she said but seemed unconcerned. "We'll recheck it in four hours next time we do vitals. It's been a little erratic."

I didn't object because I was becoming accustomed to the pulse being all over the board due to various drugs. My average resting heart rate was 56 – which almost no one in the hospital believed, being so low – but it's been that way for 40 years. Lately, however, with various drugs, I had seen it rarely below 90. Besides that, the biopsy was negative – no cancer – so what was there to fear?

What, indeed?

I acquiesced and went to sleep.

The next night, same routine: "BP 120 over 69, pulse 139, temp 98.4, oxygen 96 percent." She looked at me expectantly.

"Stop," I said. "This is not right." I held out my arm. "Check it manually, could you please?"

She checked my wrist but could not get a good reading on the pulse. I tried it, and I couldn't either. There were a couple of beats, then some confusing impulses, and then a couple more beats. "This is wrong," I said. "I don't know what you call this, but the heart is funky."

I usually did not assert myself with the medical staff, but this seemed like the time for it. "I'm going to ask you to call the doctor," I said, "right now, please. My pulse rate should not be that rapid or that jumpy. Something is bad wrong."

See how easily I had mastered the techo-med lingo?

She made the call, and soon there followed a confusing nighttime array of technicians, heart monitors, an EKG cart, nurses, and, as I recall, a trip to an MRI or a CT scan. It is a blur to me now, but the upshot was that the condition was arrhythmia – an irregular heartbeat – caused by atrial fibrillation. A doctor explained that this was probably due to the interaction of so many different drugs for so long. The cardiologist had been made aware of it and would determine what to do in the morning.

I went to bed, eventually, wondering if there would be a morning.

There was. The cardio guy was from Syria had been in the U.S. for 20 years, had applied for citizenship, and loved America. He was soft-spoken in speech but was genuinely interested in my case. "You have a-fib," he said, "atrial fibrillation. It causes arrhythmia, a fluttering of the heartbeat."

"Is it a bad thing?" I asked. "What's the impact?"

"It's not good," he replied. "Your heart is not working to capacity, and, eventually, this could kill you. What will happen is that the inefficient pumping will allow blood clots to develop. If one develops in the wrong place, it will enter a heart valve and stop it from working."

That seemed straightforward enough. The situation was challenging but not scram-the-reactor urgent. The doctor described three or four different treatment regimens to bring it under control, the last one being something he called cardioversion. This was a new term, but I understood it referred to an electric shock.

I think they create words like that to keep the peasants from realizing what it is. "So, it's like a lobotomy," I declared.

"That's a little extreme," he said with a smile. "The cardioversion is a single electric shock administered to the heart. It should stop the arrhythmia and restore the routine pulse you are accustomed to."

"Does it work?"

He pursed his lips. "Most of the time," he equivocated. "But it's not in view in your case. I don't like using it because it can be unreliable. There are serious potential side effects; sometimes, the procedure must be repeated. But a lot of the time, repeat treatment doesn't work either."

So, we would use a particular drug regimen for two days (more drugs to fix a problem created by too many drugs – but he was the doctor, after all), and that should straighten out the heart thing.

Somewhere in here, another doctor (do you get the impression they all began to run together?) explained that the heart generates its own electrical impulse. This is within the aorta and is approximately at an 11 o'clock position concerning everything else. Normally, there is a single, strong impulse. Then, as it spreads through the heart muscle, the ventricle responds with a second impulse, giving the "lub-dub" we all know and love. When an arrhythmia occurs, she explained, the aorta becomes confused. It does the single strong impulse, but half a dozen other, lesser impulses are simultaneously generated from different locations in the aorta. This causes multiple flutters of faint heartbeats and confuses the ventricle's response.

This all sounded like black magic, but I didn't argue. I recognized she was describing what happens, not necessarily why or how it happens. I was sure I would need help to follow the why and how, even if she explained it. I was a Speech major, after all.

"So, if we use the electric shock, that's supposed to get the aorta's attention?" I asked.

"Exactly," she said with a nod. "It usually puts the aorta back on track and stops all those secondary impulses."

"Usually?"

She shrugged dismissively. "Usually. But we are not using it for you. We are using drug therapy instead. Much more reliable," she finished with a smile.

Two days later, the cardio doc arrived for his routine early morning visit. We talked over a few things; he listened to my heart, said he wanted to check some test results, and left. A few minutes later, Lynn arrived. We began our morning routine... breakfast, mail, idle discussion about our kids, local gossip, and a nap.

Two hours later, we were surprised to see the doctor back. No smile this time. "It's never a good sign when your cardio doctor visits you twice on the same day," he said. He was serious.

"I just thought you liked us," I replied.

He shook off the humor and looked out the window absently as he continued. "We have determined that cardioversion is the correct procedure," he said. "We will administer it today."

"The drugs didn't work?" I asked.

"The results are not as satisfactory as we would like." I thought, *Yeah, that would be a No.* He cleared his throat and continued to avoid eye contact. "There are some risks with cardioversion." Then, he began a list of possible side effects, and I'm sure he had memorized them for recitation. This appeared to be the legal disclaimer. There were four or five possible effects, but buried in the middle was the one that got our attention.

Lynn and I agreed later it was as though his side-effect speech was, "Blah blah blah, blah blah blah, STROKE! blah blah blah blah blah blah, blah blah." That's all we heard.

For all my tough guy persona, I think I feared stroke most of all, even more than mortality. Death was one thing – I was confident I knew what was on the other side, as well as could be known: Christian faith is a powerful thing. But I had seen the results of stroke in friends of mine. They were older, and I was approaching that older age range myself. The thought of disability of movement, and especially the slurred speech that characterized so many I knew, gave me serious pause.

I had been speaking in public since sixth grade. High school was a mélange of forensics, state speech contests, debate, and school plays. My career in sales, frequently presenting before sizable audiences, was marked by a facility managing a crowd through verbal acumen. I had also done extensive layman's preaching in church, and, with tongue in cheek, I had always claimed that when called to fill in for a regular preacher, the less notice I had, the better. Fifteen minutes' warning, and I'm good.

Once my boss asked if I would moderate a breakout session at a national conference before a large audience. "Is there a microphone involved?" I asked. "Yes," he replied. "I'm in," I confirmed, and then followed up with, "What's the topic?"

This aspect of my life being in jeopardy was more unsettling than anything that had come before.

And what would my stroke do to Lynn? Taking care of a bedridden man was not a pleasant prospect. She is an adventurous, outdoors girl who needs her travel freedom. Six months after her first knee replacement at age 60, she climbed a 14er in Colorado. (That state has more than 50 peaks over 14,000 feet in elevation, and something of a cult has built up around summiting them all.) I'm pretty sure she determined the time frame from a previous hiking trip, where she had met a woman on the trail who was climbing such a peak and had had her knee replaced barely six months earlier.

Lynn can be competitive, and I'm sure she thought: *She doesn't look so tough. If she can do it, I can do it.*

Tying her to a disabled husband was not something I wanted to subject her to. I knew she had signed up for it, just as I had 38 years earlier, with the deceptively simple phrase, "for better or for worse," but the "worse" part was now a real and genuinely fearsome prospect.

But there was nothing to do but pray and put on a brave face. With the doctor in the room, I swallowed hard.

"When do we go?" I asked.

"This afternoon," he said, looking me in the eye. "I have already ordered the procedure, and the transport people should be here shortly."

Chapter 8

~~~~~~~~~~~~~~~~~~~

Other Voices

Mary and I had just been to our family reunion in Conyers, Georgia – the one Curt and Lynn skipped with some thin excuse about a cancer diagnosis – when Lynn called and told us he had a-fib and needed electric shock treatment. Not wanting to miss the fireworks, so to speak, we stopped off in Wichita.

The cardio surgeon met us in the waiting room. Lynn asked him, in mock seriousness, "Can I be the one to push the button?"

He couldn't help but laugh, then smiled ruefully, and as he turned away for the operating room, said, "I'm gonna tell him you said that." It seemed to break the tension for the doc. For a-fib, we were out of options at that point, and he understood the consequences of failure better than anyone.

He came back 15 minutes later, and I could tell from the cat-that-ate-the-canary look on his face that the procedure had been successful. – Brudder RC

~~~~~~~~~~~~~~~~~~~

The operating room, if that was what it was, was a simple affair. A machine loomed large over me as I laid back on a bed. I was a little groggy but was only on a mild sedative for fear of aspirating in the middle of the procedure. I was awake throughout.

Until I wasn't.

It was not a lengthy procedure but made up in intensity what it lacked in duration.

I was a little surprised to discover the machine would be run by the actual cardio doc who had consulted with me; there were no technicians to operate the equipment.

I wondered what exactly the procedure entailed... and then the gun went off.

The shot hit me square in the middle of the sternum with a loud POP! It did not have the depth and timbre of a firearm but rather the cold, unexpected and terrifying snap of a large electrical charge. And so it was. I felt it through my body, knowing I jerked clear off the bed in an involuntary and unavoidable muscle spasm.

I said aloud, "Oh God!" – an exclamation I would never utter under normal circumstances.

And there was something else; stay with me here: With the impulse, there was a sudden vision of a brilliant yellow-white rectangle suspended in front of me. It was three-quarters of an inch wide and three inches tall. The edges were crisp, but the image was incredibly bright as it flashed suddenly with the electric shock. It was not a doorway, not a tunnel; there were no people around it or on the other side. It was merely that vertical rectangle suspended in front of me for a brief second.

It faded quickly and drifted away to the top right of my vision. I wondered at the block of light, and then I remember thinking distinctly: *This procedure should never be performed on any human, ever!* And then all went black, and I assume that I passed out. After that, I knew no more until I awoke in my room in the cancer ward.

I stared at the white-tiled institutional drop-ceiling for a moment before recalling where I was, then fumbled for a pulse. I found it steady, rhythmic, and deliberate. Familiar and comforting, the cardioversion had worked.

When the doctor came to visit early the following morning, I greeted him with, "You must be very proud of yourself today!" He grinned like a 14-year-old boy with a blue-ribbon heifer at the State Fair.

That morning I contemplated that somehow, besides the initial diagnosis, a death sentence for many, I had overcome the two-week window to begin chemotherapy, the catheter, and the atrial fibrillation. Not to mention that I had seen nothing short of miraculous intervention in mouth sores and the ampho-terrible chills.

Chapter 8

What was so hard about all that? I thought; but I knew that every piece had found me dancing very near the edge. I was getting a little tired of being threatened with permanent cancellation.

What I did not know was that it was about to get much worse.

Theological Contemplations

In truth, I felt a little sheepish, claiming that I suffered from Acute Myeloid Leukemia. It kills many people, but I evidenced almost no ill effects. The mouth sores were gone, the amphotericin chills had been banished, I had a clean biopsy, the a-fib was cured, and I still felt fine. On the fifth day of chemotherapy Induction, Lynn asked a nurse, "So, when is he going to get sick?" She replied, "Maybe by Day 10. Don't worry," she smiled, "it'll happen."

Happen it did, the very next day. I lived inside The Crash for a week. It included bouts of fever, headache, diarrhea, nausea, sleeplessness, widespread aching, and general discomfort. But on balance, I wouldn't call it a colossal crisis. Sure, it was no picnic, but I've had the flu worse than that. Frankly, the most challenging part was turning over in a narrow bed built for somebody two-thirds my size, managing all the tethers and tubes. *Remember Paul Tibbets.*

Nearly 12,000 Americans die from AML every year. The medical journals say that only 27 percent of AML patients will live five years past the diagnosis. For those of us who also have the FLT-3 variant, that figure drops to somewhere between 10 and 15 percent. I have no idea which side of that statistic I will be on, and I am not about to claim brashly, "I'm gonna beat this thing!" because I have no idea if I will. That's God's deal, not mine.

~~~~~~~~~~~~~~~~~~~

Other Voices

When you live in a small town, you get used to hearing rumors. So when I started hearing talk of Curt being in the hospital, I wasn't sure what to believe. Once I found it to be true, I was in shock, just like everyone else. Not seeing him at our monthly City Council meeting made things very somber. For although we did have our differences, we both have always wanted what is best for the City and the citizens who live here.

As sad as I was hearing the news, there were two things I knew for sure. (1) Curt was going to fight harder than anyone I knew to beat this. (2) Curt's devotion to God. There is nothing that God can't handle, and the faith Curt had would help him fight this. – Tyler, Mayor of Benton

~~~~~~~~~~~~~~~~~~~

We play the hand we're dealt. A couple of Old Testament figures highlight this reality.

That old boy Job had a tough time, but he accepted the challenge. While he did spend some time lodging understandable complaints with the Lord, he landed on his feet at the end. I doubt that eased his pain of loss, but it's a nice touch for the denouement. I've always wondered whether that book is historical or allegory; it seems so highly stylized and contrived that I lean toward the latter. It appears in the collection of Poetry books, along with Psalms, Proverbs, Ecclesiastes, and Song of Solomon, giving some credence to a surreal interpretation. But it's still Scripture, has always been considered Scripture, and neither Jesus nor the apostles singled it out for discounting.

At any rate, Job walked the hard road put before him.

Moses, too, saw hardship: Born into a household of fabulous wealth, forced to leave by his own action, and called to 40 years of impossible service at age 80. He, too, complained from time to time, but he still stepped up.

We do not always get to choose the trials we face; only how we face them.

I believe the only Psalm attributed to Moses is the 90th, a beautiful prayer: *Lord, You have been our dwelling place throughout all generations (verse 1).* The language soars to heaven while acknowledging the reality of life on earth: *Our days may come to seventy years, or eighty, if our strength endures; yet the best of them are but trouble and sorrow... (verse 10).*

The most informative piece I take from that work is Verse 12: *Teach us to number our days, that we may gain a heart of wisdom.* The irony, of course, is that we cannot number our days, for we do not know how many there will be. I strongly suspect that objection is born of a Westerner's mentality. We are literal people, but this is a poetic text. Perhaps a better translation – or maybe an application of this passage – would be, *Teach us that our days are numbered so that we may learn to live them wisely.*

I'm no scholar, so take that for what it's worth.

So far, I had faced several trials – they were beginning to run together, such that I found it difficult to enumerate them – but now things were looking up. I was past the Induction crash. It was time to relax because I would return home in a few days.

And then my spleen blew up.

Guam, 1944

They watched the carrier-based fighter come in for a landing. As the pilot touched down, he wrestled the small plane into a yaw, squalling the tires in protest, and shuddered to a stop near the refueling area. The gas detail raced the fuel truck to his side. Dad gave the plane a quick once-over, confirmed his suspicions, and spoke to the pilot.

"You've got a bad landing gear, Sir," he said. "It's about to fold up on you, and you did a good job landing the way you did. Taxi it over to the maintenance area, Sir, and we can get you fixed up in no time."

"Not now, chief," he said. "I've gotta get back in the air. I can take off the same way I came in, holding the gear down by putting sideways pressure on it."

"Well, yessir, you can," Dad admitted, "but it could fold up on you. We'd be glad to look at it."

"Look, chief," the pilot countered, "my carrier is headed for Pearl Harbor. Two weeks of R&R are waiting for me, and I'm not missing that ship!"

"Yes, Sir!" the chief replied and snapped a salute. The crew finished with the fuel in record time, retracted the hoses, and watched him power down the coral strip almost sideways, tires shrieking until he rotated off the runway.

The incident (because it was a single-seat, carrier-based fighter) probably involved a Grumman F4F Wildcat or the later F6F Hellcat model. The way the wheels retract into the fuselage suggests a Wildcat; holding one out with lateral pressure would be more likely with the Wildcat design. It would have been far too easy when Dad was still living to enquire about these details, but I never asked. The date when it happened would suggest whether there was a significant enemy engagement going on at the time. The type of aircraft – which Dad surely would have remembered – could indicate which carrier was involved, and the rotation back to Pearl Harbor would place the event in history. It might even have been possible to identify the pilot involved.

I should have asked. We tend to assume that life will go on forever and that no one will be interested in our stories. Neither is true.

We will never know how or whether that aviator got down onto his carrier, but I'd be interested. There was a man with an appreciation of his situation, confidence in his abilities, and a focus on his priorities.

Chapter 9

Caring Bridge Journal, July 20 – July 25, 2022

July 20

Chemo Day 26. Beginning to discuss discharging from hospital, but cannot leave until the lung fungus is gone, or at least under better control. Also, all 3 blood levels (RB, WB and platelets) need to be able to hold their own. While strong, they do not yet have the full numbers needed.

Also there is swelling in the lowers, a holdover from all this IV treatment. That will take time to fix but does not necessarily have to be done in-patient.

I walked hallway laps twice today, and per the Sweatcoin app that's about 1800 ft. Brudder RC was here and supervised one of those outings. See photo.

Here is a good one for remaining physically fit:

Jeremiah 12:5 If thou hast run with the footmen, and they have wearied thee, then how canst thou contend with horses? and if in the land of peace, wherein thou trustedst, they wearied thee, then how wilt thou do in the swelling of Jordan?

Enjoy your evening, and in spite of the above verse, perhaps you should remain in the A/C for tonight. Or this week. Curt

July 21

Chemo Day 27. Pancakes and sausage for breakfast, appetite is coming back.

MRI this morning at cardio Doc's request; no issues except for the arrhythmia which has been dealt with. I think he wanted to see if some issue was responsible for that condition.

Cancer Doc: You are prolly going to be dismissed next week. The meds are being changed over to orals rather than drips. Timing of release depends on progress against the lung fungus. Still have significant swelling of legs and feet due to water retention… that's a slow battle over the next month prolly, requiring some exercise.

Physical exercise would be extraordinarily good at this point.

With the Induction phase largely done, next phase is Consolidation, which means chemo one week per month, prolly out-patient. Woo hoo.

We will see this through. I cannot imagine navigating this rough water without your prayers. It has sort of changed my perspective on the nature of the church.

Ecclesiastes 7:8. Better is the end of a thing than the beginning thereof: and the patient in spirit is better than the proud in spirit.

Curt

July 22

Chemo Day 28. Appetite is up, blood levels are up. Swelling in legs and feet is up... yeah it's just water retention but that does not mean it can be ignored.

Lung fungus continues its retreat under heavy antibiotic push. (But remember the army of the Third Reich was in retreat after January 1945 but didn't cave for another 4 months.)

We have at least two days of fungus treatment remaining followed by a CT scan Monday, which should say it's all clear. If the fungus reads the same script. I walked the halls with my Mobility Aide this morning, showing off the camo kilt. Would like to get out again but am tethered to the juice bar and the elevated feet. Grrr.

Habakkuk 3:19 The LORD God is my strength, and he will make my feet like hinds' feet, and he will make me to walk upon mine high places. Curt

July 23

Chemo Day 29. This hospital bed will do amazing contortions but the cool stuff is controlled on the outside of the safety panel where the inmate can't see what's what. Friendly nurse applied a work-around: A pair of adhesive EKG electrode pads to two of the switches I can't see. By reaching over the rail I can touch those to raise and lower my feet, and in that way can elevate those swollen appendages for proper rest. It's a tilt-a-whirl machine. It promotes independence, and because I am up every hour bc of that blankety blank water pill, I can manage my own schedule.

I'm on something like 5 grams a day of potassium, which prolly has to do with kidney function. It comes in large horse pills 2 at a time, 3 times a day, and each one is a Heimlich maneuver in the making. Solution: Day nurse dissolved the pills in water (they reduce to hundreds of tiny time release globules) and drizzled it into a ration of applesauce, then I stir it up and eat the applesauce. Problem solved. Just don't crunch the gritty parts; chase it with water and swallow it whole.

Interestingly, we have had to train each shift on that protocol.

Lynn walked me this morning (hallway laps), and while I would like to sit up in a chair, I have confined myself to the bed for the elevated feet thing.

Acts 3:8. And he leaping up stood, and walked, and entered with them into the temple, walking, and leaping, and praising God.

Walking and leaping is a good thing! Curt

July 24

Chemo Day 30 ALMOST THE LAST DAY. This is July 24, day 33 of hospitalization. Tomorrow Monday is probably the actual day of dismissal (though that could change) but I suspect there will be enough activity then that I may not have time for a final journal entry.

Chapter 9

I cannot adequately express my heartfelt appreciation to you who have prayed, commented and followed this journal. I am quite convinced I have seen the results of your prayers, and I am quite convinced I needed them.

There was a Star Trek TV episode where Kirk, Spock and McCoy faced 3 deadly aliens (all miniskirted girls, for some reason). Each alien was programmed for a particular target and could not harm the others. Kirk always led, of course, and when the alien leader intoned "I am for Kirk," he was uncharacteristically taken aback. He stepped to the rear and said, "Gentlemen, I think I need your help."

Not that my theology comes from Gene Roddenberry, but that scene is an appropriate word picture of the necessity and value of the church interceding for one another.

Next moves: All the pharmaceuticals (and they are legion) have been converted to orals so that I can sustain them at home. We have two weeks now of relative calm while the antibiotics finish their course and get purged from the system. Then comes the Consolidation Phase.

The Induction Phase, now finished, refers to the initial hospitalization with a week of chemo and 3 weeks of observation and recovery. Per the Onc Doc, if we simply stopped all treatments at this point the leukemia would recur full strength in a month. Ergo, we now enter the Consolidation Phase, a four month period with chemotherapy one week out of four.

Those next rounds of chemo will not be as shocking to the system as the initial, but they are still designed to kill bone marrow activity, and thus white blood cells, red blood cells, and platelets. Which leaves the patient vulnerable to bad actors. Further, there is no predicting how I will respond to the next chemos; Maybe these are out-patient, maybe some days will require in-patient treatment. I would dearly love to have a planned schedule, but that ain't how it works.

Proverbs 16:9. The mind of a man plans his way, but the Lord directs his steps.

I know, it's not KJV… must be the meds. Curt

July 25

I got a call a little bit ago saying that Curt was being transferred to CICU. He couldn't breathe and his BP was low. 95/57 right now. He's on oxygen and will get another unit of blood. This is all quite a surprise as we thot we were going home today. I wish I had more to tell you but once again I'm asking you to approach the throne boldly on behalf of Curt.

I'm counting on you. Lynn

July 25
Lynn's 2nd status report

Curt will go to surgery soon. They think a ruptured spleen but could be other issues. Please pray for him. You all know what to pray. "So whether you eat or drink or whatever you do, do it all to the glory of God." May this too, be for his glory. Lynn

July 25
Lynn's 3rd status report
Surgery was successful. More later
Praise God from whom all blessings flow
Thank you for praying

Inflection Point 4 – The Night of the Exploding Spleen

Two weeks later, on a Sunday night, I was ready to go home. The fungus was being treated with a drug; all the intravenous drugs had been converted to oral pills to facilitate home consumption. I would leave for two weeks and then return for the first round of the Consolidation phase.

Earlier that day, I had written this on Caring Bridge:

Chemo Day 30 ALMOST THE LAST DAY. This is July 24, day 33 of hospitalization. Tomorrow Monday is probably the actual day of dismissal (though that could change) but I suspect there will be enough activity then that I may not have time for a final journal entry.

I concluded the post with this passage, which was eerily prescient: *Proverbs 16:9. The mind of a man plans his way, but the Lord directs his steps.*

Well... not so fast on the dismissal thing.

Everything was fine until I got into bed, took a deep breath, and my eyes flew wide open as something grated inside. I sat up and felt sharp pains throughout my chest.

Heart attack? Not exactly. No shortness of breath, clammy skin, charley horse, or left arm pain. But pain there was, and in seconds it became excruciating.

Chapter 9

I explained to Lynn days later that all the stars of Heaven had fallen from the sky, landed inside my chest, and were all made of broken glass. I could not sit still; I could not move; I could not breathe; I could not swallow; I could not move without severe, stabbing, shockingly sharp pain. After the danger passed, and compassionate soulmate that she was, she merely rolled her eyes.

Weeks later, I was able to debrief this event with Nurse K. She explained that she had met me briefly when I had first arrived in the cancer ward, but she was pregnant then and left to deliver her child. So this night was her first back from maternity leave.

As it happened, another nurse had failed to show up for duty that night, and a half-dozen patients were redistributed among the remaining staff. I was given to K as light duty because it was her first night back, my last night in, and there was confidence that I would need no attention. I was going home the following morning.

"I looked in on you at 9:00 p.m.," K reported. "You were sitting on the edge of the bed, hunched over, complaining of pain. I asked you to rate the pain, and you said, 'Ten.'

"I didn't know what to make of that," she said. "I didn't know you, and the self-reported pain level is always a guess. I've had patients who insist they are 'Twelve on a scale of ten!' and then a few minutes later are sound asleep. So I gave you a laxative and left to deal with another patient.

"An hour later, I came back to take vitals and you were curled up on the bed in a fetal position. I thought, 'Good, maybe he's asleep, and I can get the vitals without waking him.' But you woke up and said your pain was maybe six or seven. That sounded better, but your oxygen was only 82 percent, and your BP was 80 over 40. That was bad."

At that point, K called the charge nurse, J, who offered me Sprite and Tylenol. I accepted both but wanted neither. The entire chest cavity felt filled with blood and gas, broken shards of glass grated against one another; the Sprite would make it worse, and the Tylenol would be no match for it. I was attempting to belch but could not make it happen.

While K and J discussed this, the BP suddenly dropped to 60 over 30. "In the nurse squad room," K later explained, "we call that '60 over Dead.' Almost nobody survives that. Your pulse also dropped to 30, and I immediately called for a 'Rapid.'"

A Rapid Response is hitting the panic button. K dialed a code on her cell phone – like an internal hospital 9-1-1 – and the room filled with people in less than two minutes.

My recollection of that night is fuzzy, dimly sensed through an angry red curtain of agony. K explained that over a dozen people responded to her call: A cardiac doctor, two ICU nurses, an EKG technician, every nurse from the cancer ward, a chaplain, and others. I heard someone on the telephone, urgent and agitated. Lab coats and scrubs entered and left.

"What – is – wrong – with – me?" I grated out. Talking was a new experience in pain, but so was everything else. How long could this possibly last?

But apparently, I retained some vestigial sense of humor. K told me that with everyone looking at me, I raised a hand to point at her: "You – did this – to me!" I accused.

It was probably bad timing for a laugh line. K told me later that everyone suddenly turned to look at her, expressions serious, questioning what she had done. "Wait!" she exclaimed in a panic. "He's joking! They tell me he does this all the time! I didn't do anything to him!"

She was still employed two months later, so I suppose it blew over. I apologized to her all the same.

Chapter 9

A cart showed up to carry me to Cardiac ICU. I saw it and groaned. A transfer to the transport cart is made by first rolling the body to one side, up against the side rail of the bed. A sheet is tucked beneath the patient, then the body is physically rolled onto the back and against the other rail. The sheet is extended; the body is rolled onto the back again. Four nurses grab the corners of the sheet and drag the patient across to the transport cart.

The experience of rolling from one side to another with a chest full of broken glass cannot adequately be described. For once in my life, I screamed. Not just once, but as many times as seemed reasonable.

Lynn was summoned from home at 12:30 a.m. On the phone, a nurse told her, "You don't need to come. Curt says to wait till morning."

Another nurse's voice in the background, shouting, came through the receiver to Lynn. "No! You need to come now!"

She did.

I have a few snatches of memory; I have no idea where the events occurred or their sequence.

I was rolled again as a solid board was shifted underneath me. This would have been for an x-ray, and I'm pretty sure I made obstreperous vocalizations again.

At some point, a doctor told me that a bladder sonogram had been ordered. *So what?* I thought. *Just make the hurt go away!*

Another snatch of a conversation: There was blood in the bladder. "What does that mean?" I gasped.

"Probably a ruptured spleen," he said casually, as though discussing whether there would be ranch dressing available in the cafeteria today. "If so, we'll just take it out." I saw him shrug. "You don't need it anyway."

I had questions, but it was too much work to ask. *Doesn't the spleen do something? If not, why did God put it there? Why did it rupture? What does that have to do with all the broken glass?*

"But we don't know if it's the spleen yet," he said, and I think he thought this would be reassuring. "We'll have to look around and see what's broken. But, whatever it is," he finished confidently, "we'll fix it."

I was too far gone to argue. Did I sleep? Pass out? Did morphine take me away? Somehow the night passed because they told me later that the surgery had not been performed until 10:00 a.m.

Weeks later, another doctor explained that blood outside the vascular system is highly abrasive. "It feels like sharp stabbing pains," he said. "So, when you had a little loose in the bladder, it caused great pain. Also, as it filled your chest cavity, it would have felt like grating, stabbing wounds. And besides that," he added, "when your abdomen is involved, your brain cannot localize the origin of pain. You don't know where it's coming from, so it feels like it's coming from all over." That described my experience perfectly.

And then, sometime in the night: A nurse in my face, left side, urgently shouting: "Stay with me! Stay with me! Stay with me!" Lynn told me later that this was in the wee hours of the morning, well before the surgery, when there was, shall we say, heightened concern about my longevity. Or lack thereof.

While the nurse was shouting at me, I had a vision – and this is quite graphic, etched into my memory – of a white index card, four inches square, in front of my face. The center was bright white, and the edges were disintegrating, turning to snow like a TV channel with no signal. I could not see the corners of the card or the edges because of the deterioration. I knew this was not real, but it was a real vision, clear and distinct. It seemed of utmost importance to focus on the card.

"Stay with me! Stay with me, Curt!"

Somehow this meant I must remain in the center of that card and not slip off to the edge. I ground out words slowly: "I – do not – want – to stay – with you!"

"No! Stay with me! Count backward from ten!"

Chapter 9

Someone else was there, right side, bothering me. *Can't you leave me alone?* I thought. Shaking my shoulders, slapping my face, my chest, my arms, hard. *Why would you treat me this way? Can't you leave me alone?*

The bottom right corner of the white card was disintegrating. The snow crept inexorably toward the center of the card. Somehow, I had a strong feeling that at the bottom right corner was peace; I should slip off to that corner. It would be so easy, and I found myself sliding in that direction.

But the voice, frantic, had said to stay with her. There was an urgency to it, an imperative. What could possibly be that important? Just a few minutes in the bottom right corner would be so good. The pull was overwhelming.

But no... she had said... what? *Count backward from ten.* "Four — three — two — one," I ground out. It took all my strength. I heard my voice, and it was the sound of gravel. It hurt to speak. From someplace I wondered what contrary nature made me start at four instead of ten in a situation like this.

And what exactly was this situation, anyway? The physical agony was excruciating, but from somewhere, I knew the battle was also mental. Or spiritual.

"Stay with me!"

The corner beckoned, but no, she had been insistent, and it must be of critical importance for her to speak to me like that. The shaking and slapping continued from the other side, making me angry and impatient, but it also seemed somehow important. As much as anything, the physical harassment pushed me back to the center of the card.

"Eight — seven — six — five!" It hurt, and my words were distorted and distant. The center of the card; stay in the center. Don't look at the bottom right corner. It beckoned, but now it seemed somehow... wrong. It would be so easy to go there and peaceful... but wrong. Dangerously wrong, frighteningly wrong. Stay in the center. Stay in the center. Stay in...

And then nothing further. I do not know if the bottom right corner of that ephemeral index card in my vision was unconsciousness or death, but it was one or the other. I can still recall the overwhelming pull.

Through the night in the intensive care unit, it was Lynn and a nurse who had been on either side of me, trying to keep me from slipping into unconsciousness. They spent the morning hours there; Lynn said they lost me three times, unconscious, and each time got me back by frantic shake-and-shout.

They saved my life.

Of the spleen surgery, I have no recollection. Still, there are snatches of video and audio, probably from just before the operating room: A sudden, brief impression of lights in the ceiling going by fast – the distant rumble of the cart's wheels. Many people around the moving bed. A few bumps and shakes, more stabbing pain. There was so much of it, and it had been so continuous that it dominated everything.

A strong male voice: "Can we get in here ahead of you? I don't think this one can wait."

And then nothing.

I learned later that the surgery was successful. The surgeon had been summoned from home early that morning to perform my emergency splenectomy. The operation at 10:00 a.m. was 13 hours after the onset of symptoms, so my guess is the mountain of discomfort I had felt the night before was from the rupture, but it had taken the medicos several hours to determine the location.

They extracted two liters of blood from my chest cavity during the procedure. The body only holds about five liters; a 40% loss is in the fatal range. They pumped in replacement units as fast as they could.

Afterward, doctors discovered a ball of Fusarium had attached itself to the spleen. Filtering impurities is the spleen's job; apparently, it had tried valiantly and been overwhelmed by the invader.

Happy news, the patient survived. And that should have been that, but it wasn't.

The next threat showed up barely an hour later.

Theological Contemplations

It was not an emergency until it was, and then it was all hands on deck.

The ruptured spleen could only be called a near-death experience. Maybe I could make the cover of a grocery store check-out line rag with this? Is there any money in that? Probably not... I think those are reserved for pretty, divorced Hollywood people who are having someone else's baby. I don't think I qualify.

Since that eventful night, I have contemplated what went right. Almost nothing went wrong, though there were several points where we could easily have run off the rails, in which case I would now be unconcerned with the post-game analysis. Instead, you would be clucking your tongues ("Too bad for him... what was his name, anyway?") and going about your unenlightened lives.

Doctor A, the infectious disease specialist, insisted that a one-degree fever meant Something Important. To me, that sort of thing had always suggested there was merely a lightweight infection being fought off by the immune system

. In normal conditions, taking Ibuprofen or equivalent would suppress the fever and probably also suppress the defense mechanism. I have always thought, therefore, that one should avoid treating the fever until it becomes too uncomfortable. Let the body do its work unimpeded by mere creature comfort.

But the doctor immediately came to a different and more informed conclusion, which is, incidentally, what she is paid for. She recognized that my immune system was compromised to the point where it could not effectively fight the infection. There was defensive activity, which was why there was a fever, but the body was no match for it. External intervention was required, which took the form of a biopsy, an IV drip, and a referral to the Mayo Clinic.

Jesus pointed out that in the economy of the Kingdom of God, the one who has demonstrated faithfulness in a few things (small things) will be given responsibility over many things (big things). *(Luke 16:10)*. This is a lesson worth learning. In my case, it was a lifesaver.

Doctor A was a character. At a petite 5'2" and sporting a new outfit every day – I kid you not, every day – she was a commanding figure. She was pleasant, loquacious, personable, and firmly focused on patient care, primarily patient survival.

Weeks after this event, I asked her about the Fusarium fungus. "Isn't there some test we can do to determine if it's still active?"

"It is not active now," she replied, "and there is not a good test to determine what its status is. But it is still in your system. Look," she said, "we are going to keep you safe from the Fusarium. That thing is a killer. You may die from leukemia; that's not my department. But you are not going to die from an infection on my watch. So take the pills I prescribe, and don't argue!"

"Okay, you win!" I laughed. Such passion and straight talk. I loved it.

We would probably never have had that conversation if she had ignored the one-degree fever. As it was, we almost didn't anyway.

In her line of business, it does not pay to overlook the details.

Chapter 9

~~~~~~~~~~~~~~~~~~~~

Other Voices

What a journey of faith and suspense this has been, apropos of a Hollywood thriller. And the good guy wins, as we all knew he would. But it was a real cliffhanger from the get-go. Curt's upbeat attitude kept many of us from realizing how close to the cliff he was, which is a real tribute to his monumental determination to face this trial with faith and courage.

Through what can aptly be termed an arduous and harrowing ordeal, we all learned... wait for it... Curt truly is a tough guy. Even his oncologist used those words. – Brudder RC

~~~~~~~~~~~~~~~~~~~~

Despite my effort to get her fired on the Night of the Exploding Spleen, Nurse K rose to the occasion without hesitation or timidity. Were it not for her immediate decision to call the Rapid, that night would have been much shorter for one of us and much longer for the other.

For her, it will no doubt be a career highlight.

Several weeks after the event, we had the opportunity to discuss it at length. She was on duty, and I was concerned about her schedule. "I'm sorry to take your time," I said. "This happened a long time ago, and I don't want to interfere with your other patients."

"No problem," she said with a laugh. "I have told this story a hundred times and don't mind going through it again. Nobody needs me right now, anyway."

It was a signal event in her nursing career. It would not have been a happy memory if she had not acted with needful alacrity.

*****

Was it necessary to have 15 people sprinting through hallways, converging on my room to ponder one case?

Who knows?

No one knows, which is precisely the point. I spent much of my career working with emergency responders. Universally, they have agreed that their shifts are spent in tedious routine maintenance until they get a call. At that point, all they know is what the dispatcher relays: Structure fire; a highway wreck with multiple victims; a man with a gun; choking victim. The only proper response is a fast response with overwhelming resources.

In about 2009, I was at a national emergency communications trade show in Orlando. There was an evening social event at a piano bar three blocks from the host hotel. About a hundred of us made the walk; virtually everyone in that business had some degree of training and experience with emergency medical treatment.

One of our conferees, about age 60, collapsed on the sidewalk in the darkening evening. A small crowd formed; professionals established a perimeter to allow space to work. A couple of flashlights appeared. Those near the fallen man leaped into action; it is a truism that first responders foam at the mouth for a good roadside emergency.

Two people checked for pulse and respiration and began CPR. It was probably a heart attack.

Ric and I approached the group. I had known Ric for 20 years; he was charmingly direct, opinionated, and un-subtle. "Hey!" he called out. "Has anyone called 9-1-1 yet?" Several faces turned, looking sheepish and guilty.

"I'll take that as a No!" he shouted. Then, pointing to one of our group, he said, "You, Sir. Please call 9-1-1. Tell them the name of the club; we're right outside. Tell them it's a medical emergency, we suspect a heart attack, and give them a brief description of the vic."

As the man did so, Ric shook his head and scowled. Then, he lowered his voice and said, "These guys are nuts. We're all Johnny-on-the-Spot, supposed to be professionals and know how to handle a simple emergency, but nobody thinks to call 9-1-1." He scoffed. "Nobody here has a crash kit, and probably nobody has looked into Florida state law to see if there is a Good Samaritan statute. All they gotta do is call 9-1-1." He scanned the busy street and the many night spots within view. "Downtown in the tourist strip? There's probably an EMT station two minutes away, waiting for something to do."

The siren of an approaching ambulance drowned out the last of his comments.

"I'd make that 60 seconds," I said.

*****

At St. Francis, the cancer ward on 7-North has over the years developed a close relationship with the Cardiac Intensive Care Unit (CICU). The personnel in both units know one another, and there seems to be much mutual respect. So when K and J saw my plunging blood pressure and pulse rate, and K called the Rapid, the natural response was to dispatch me to CICU.

In my experience, any work area that hands off a problem to another must provide an attendant explanation, query resources, and request assistance. This takes time, as the receiving group balances the urgency of the need with their capacity to accept it.

Between 7-North and CICU, this transfer was accomplished with zero delay. The informal relationships between professionals on both sides proved invaluable. Seconds counted. When my punishing ride on a tortuous cart ended at intensive care, they were ready for me. I was utterly oblivious to the activity that no doubt swarmed about me; I have no recollection of entering the ward. I suppose I was unconscious at the time.

The CICU reaction was fast, competent, and overwhelming.

Likewise, the call to Lynn with the shouted, "No! You need to come now!" and the nurse in my face with the urgent, "Stay with me!" commands.

When things need to happen big, they need to happen big.

Maybe it's their training. I have no doubt that everyone in scrubs that night had contemplated this type of situation before, and most had probably been involved in some very like it. When the balloon went up, they knew what to do and what to expect. A young nurse took urgent action on the first night back from maternity leave. A false or premature panic call on her part would have her facing a harsh supervisory review, probably career-affecting.

She had already thought about the consequences of failure – both of acting and not acting – and, while probably not comfortable, knew exactly what to do and when to do it.

*****

Jonah, the Old Testament prophet, was a guy who had failed to prepare ahead of time. When he got the call from God to go to Nineveh with an unpopular message, he lost no time taking passage on a ship in the Med.

A quick check of any Bible atlas will show he went in the opposite direction of the Lord's intended destination. No surprise to God, but the ship's crew probably didn't think much of it. Or, for that matter, the whale.

Nineveh was the biggest news around at that time, a haven of impurity and godlessness. Any devout Jew knew this, and it should not have been a shock to receive God's command to preach a sermon to them. Or maybe Jonah *had* prepared; he had merely prepared to run away.

By contrast, the "sons of Issachar" *understood the times and knew what Israel should do (1 Chronicles 12:32).*

Chapter 9

The elements critical to survival on this night seemed to be an awareness of the situation and the willingness to act decisively. Assess with perspective and execute with determination.

South Pacific, ca. 1944

James Michener's Pulitzer Prize-winning *Tales of the South Pacific* (Bantam Books, 1946) is an historical fiction on which the Broadway play of similar name was based. It includes a chapter called "The Milk Run," the story of World War II fighter/bomber pilot Bus Adams, shot down during a routine patrol. In Adams' telling, a Milk Run is a mission with little enemy opposition. Pilots expect it to be more a sightseeing trip than a combat assignment; but on this day, his Douglas SBD Dauntless dive bomber was hit by a lucky anti-aircraft shot.

He went into the water a few hundred yards from an enemy shore, and Japanese guns opened up on him.

As he floated in a tiny life raft, Bus Adams' companions overhead set up aerial cover for him. They circled his location and strafed enemy troops who targeted him. When they ran low on fuel, they were relieved by other units, one after another. The admiral, advised of the situation, ordered all assets available to rescue Adams. "Our planes are expendable," he proclaimed. "Our pilots are not!"

In an event lasting most of the day, some 100 Allied aircraft, including a PBY, U.S. Navy and Marine aviators, New Zealand fighter planes, and two PT boats were involved in the rescue. The PBY and one P-40 fighter were lost to enemy fire.

The entire operation to rescue a single pilot disrupted planned invasion schedules and cost U.S. taxpayers $600,000. "But it's sure worth every cent of the money," the fictional Adams said, "if you happen to be that pilot."

That story came to mind after the splenectomy as I surveyed the hundreds of thousands (millions?) of dollars in the equipment and staffing of CICU. What a great place is America!

I was living a good story. But it lasted only a short time before the next emergency.

Chapter 10

Caring Bridge Journal, July 25 – July 29, 2002

July 25

Lynn's 4th status report

I've called on you all so much the last 24 hrs and 34 days but once again I'm asking. Curt's kidneys have shut down and he's going on dialysis. It looks bleak but I've said this before and he has pulled thru. It's in utter contrast from an hour ago when the splenectomy was successful. This all leads me to believe this is a battle in the heavenly's. Would you pray "without ceasing" with me? I can't thank you all enough. Lynn

July 26

Lynn's status report, hospital stay day 35

Curt seems better this morning but as we know from yesterday things can change quickly. Thank you all for praying. Curt is intubated so communication is frustrating especially for him. Why didn't we practice hand signals when we were up on the cancer ward and had all that time!! And if they take that tube out today I'm sure I'm gonna hear about it!

Curt is on gentle dialysis which means it's over a 2 day stretch instead of a couple hours. So his kidneys have to start working or we have some tough decisions to make. My heart is broken and I'm so very sad. But still my hope is built on nothing less than Jesus' blood and righteousness. I dare not trust the sweetest frame but wholly lean on Jesus' name.

July 27

Lynn's status report, hospital stay day 36

I must thank you all for praying for Curt. He's a little better today than yesterday. And it makes so much difference to me knowing that you all are out there, supporting, loving and praying for us. "Be humble, and gentle; be patient, bearing with one another in love." You all have carried us in love this far and I am humbled by that and grateful to God. It's a testimony to God's goodness and your faithfulness to love and pray for us. A grateful thank you to you all.

July 27

Chemo Day 33. Greetings from Cardiac ICU. It has been a whirlwind from "Going Home" (think Dvorak, if musically inclined) to "make a new plan, Stan" (Paul Simon).

Sometime around 900p on Sunday night the spleen ruptured, began to fill the bladder and other available internal cavities, and they did emergency surgery to remove it and cast it into outer darkness where there is wailing and gnashing of teeth. The spleen is a wimp. Fortunately the patient moaning and whining went along with it.

Now we are trying to find a combination of dialysis equipment and cocktails that will allow management of BP and kidney function and pulse rate so that we may return to the main event, which at one point was leukemia.

One rabbit trail after another.

I'm sure there is more I should say but the above is confusing enough.

Specific prayer: To find that combination of equipment settings and drugs that allow us to return to the leukemia treatment.

Chin up! It's kind of cool seeing all the machines at work. Curt!

July 27

Curt's big brudder RC here, doing this post. Lynn is tired, and Curt is doing fine, but very tired. Here are some of the details. First, the kidney function appears to me to be on the mend, fairly good output this afternoon and the charge nurse is happy with that. The ruptured spleen repair appears not to be an issue, have not heard the docs talk about it much but appears to be under control and healing OK. Most vitals are stable and OK, with the exception of hemoglobin. Running at 6.8 now and had two pints of blood already, one more pint going in now, as their target is 7.0 or above on the ICU wing. We know that normal is up higher than that. A few more details, the medicine to stimulate the kidneys was administered this afternoon at about the same time Marva the marvelous appeared on the floor to do some housekeeping. Marva swung into the room and did some housecleaning of her own there with another of her heaven-sent prayer sessions. We are attributing the kidneys starting to work to that prayer of hers, as much as the medicine.

The mouth sores are well under control or gone. Curt can eat with no issue, although his appetite is low. Overall, my assessment is that Curt is very tired but in no distress and all indications are that all the immediate concerns are under control. His legs are still swollen a bit, but the doc says that will take care of itself when the kidneys kick into full function. Curt was fairly animated this morning, and in my opinion wore himself out chatting and quipping with me, the staff, and the docs. Probably overdid it and that's what made him so tired this afternoon and evening. Obviously there is still the long-term leukemia issue which will require chemotherapy, but that is not an issue for the next several days.

Chapter 10

Thanks so much to all of you who are holding Curt and the family up in prayer; that's one of the great blessings we have in that room. Cannot say enough good things about the staff and the doctors that are attending to Curt, absolutely top-notch first class care in my opinion.

July 28
Big Brudder RC here again. Quiet night. Kidneys still working very well so no current discussion of any further need for dialysis, vitals OK, hemoglobin is 7.8 so no need for more blood. Sleeping much of the time. Doing well enough that the thinking is to move out of cardiac ICU later today and back to a "normal" room in the cancer wing where he started. The doc consortium consensus is to get him out of bed this afternoon to at least sit in a chair for a few minutes. Legs are still swollen, getting wrapped with ace bandages now, so there's a prayer target. Another prayer target today would be to relieve the nausea that seems to come with almost any food ingestion. Drugs help, but still there occasionally. Thanks so much for all the supporting prayers through this process. :-) RC for Lynn

July 28
This is Big Brudder RC with another update for Thursday, July 28 coming up on 7 PM. A fairly uneventful day, PTL! Curt is tired and slept most of the day, is in good spirits when he is awake, but still weak although slowly gaining strength. Kidneys are still working fine; all the vitals were fine today. He is essentially off most of the heavy duty medication that one gets in an ICU room. The rest is mostly routine meds. So the hospitalist said he's ready to move out of ICU (that's a good indicator right there!) to his previous room, except that 7north (the cancer wing) is full. One of the nurses said most of the hospital is full. I suggested they try the maternity ward, which prompted a pregnant pause……. All in all, things appear to be better.

Very little nausea this afternoon and we had a cup of chicken broth and some bread this evening which he so far is tolerating OK. Legs are still swollen, not much change there yet. He stood up this afternoon, gracefully pirouetted and lowered himself into a chair, all with the help of four nurses. It only took two to get him back from the chair into the bed. He sat up for about an hour and a half in the chair but dozed most of that time. All in all, I believe he is slowly gaining strength and there does not seem to be any immediate issue on the horizon. Thanks again to everyone for your caring and praying. I feel like we're on the tip of a mountain with a huge prayer support base under us. :-) Brudder RC

July 29
Lynn's status report, hospital stay day 38

I'll start out with a heartfelt thank you to you all. It's an incredible experience to go thru something this difficult yet with this tremendous bedrock of love and support. Thank you.

Curt got moved back up to 7North last night, the cancer unit, which is a positive thing. That means he stabilized enough to not have to be monitored continuously down in ICU. I think the idea now is for him to get strong enough to go home. He's pretty weak right now and sleeps a lot but he needs to heal so that's a good thing.

I'm so grateful to you all. Lynn

July 29

Chemo Day 35. Funny how I never thought a move to the cancer ward would be an upgrade. I moved back here from Cardiac ICU last night.

If you ever have the opportunity for a ruptured spleen I would urge you to pass. Every cavity above the waist was jammed with blood or gas. I'm not sure how they determined the spleen was at fault, but once they did, it was removed for immediate relief. I think they also drained off 2 liters of blood; your system capacity is only 5, so some would consider that significant. (Maybe my numbers are right, maybe not.)

I was within 12 hours of dismissal when the rupture started. Timing is sort of important.

RC & Mary were a big help; they are back to Colorado now. Some have commented on his posts. He is an electrical engineer accustomed to sorting through, identifying and summarizing salient points of information. He also thinks he is as clever as I in communicating situation details while retaining an upbeat and optimistic outlook. And I think he is actually better.

I am optimistic but we are still a step at a time. The spleen thing really paused the progress and we have to make that back up. That means eating (appetite or no) and getting out to walk (strength or no). So those are the prayer requests.

1 Samuel 14:27 ...he put forth the end of the rod that was in his hand, and dipped it in an honeycomb, and put his hand to his mouth; and his eyes were enlightened. Curt

July 29

Lynn's 2nd status report

Curt has had a lot of trouble with nausea, belching, and eating. He had an X-ray earlier today and he's now down for a CT scan. They suspect a bowel blockage. He's been so strong thru all this but I can see him wearing down. And now the littlest thing makes me nervous too. I've called on you all so many times. Once more again please. I'm so thankful for you all. Lynn

Chapter 10

Inflection Point 5 – Kidney Shutdown

July 25 Lynn issued four Caring Bridge posts early in the morning, beginning with the call she received just after midnight, and they tell the story:

I got a call a little bit ago saying that Curt was being transferred to CICU. He couldn't breathe, and his BP was low. 95/57 right now. He's on oxygen and will get another unit of blood. This is all quite a surprise as we thot we were going home today. I wish I had more to tell you but once again I'm asking you to approach the throne boldly on behalf of Curt. I'm counting on you. Lynn

Curt will go to surgery soon. They think a ruptured spleen but could be other issues. Please pray for him. You all know what to pray. "So, whether you eat or drink or whatever you do, do it all to the glory of God." May this too, be for his glory.

Surgery was successful. More later

Praise God from whom all blessings flow

Thank you for praying

And then, suddenly:

I've called on you all so much the last 24 hrs and 34 days but once again I'm asking. Curt's kidneys have shut down and he's going on dialysis. It looks bleak but I've said this before and he has pulled thru. It's in utter contrast from an hour ago when the splenectomy was successful. This all leads me to believe this is a battle in the heavenly's. Would you pray "without ceasing" with me? I can't thank you all enough. Lynn

Acute renal failure is nothing to take lightly. In my case, the kidneys had been weakened by the plunging blood pressure the night before. The brain considers that its function trumps that of a mere peripheral activity (such as filtering and eliminating toxic waste products) and pinches down blood supply to everything but itself.

As we understood from the nephrologist after the fact, the outer layer of the kidney contains about a million tiny filters called nephrons. Each has a screen that prevents things like proteins and red/white blood cells from being excreted. A system of tiny tubes passes approved items (water, minerals, nutrients) to an accompanying blood vessel for return to the body. In contrast, the non-approved waste items are eventually routed to the bladder.

This sounded a lot like how the septic tank worked back on the farm: laterals, storage tank, and whatnot.

When the BP suddenly dropped, blood flow to the kidneys (and everything else except the brain) was commensurately reduced. As a result, those microscopic tubular structures began to collapse for want of blood supply. If they remained collapsed for too long, they would never be able to re-open.

Sort of like the starship *Enterprise* that time they lost the dilithium crystals. The matter-antimatter reactors went cold and could not be restarted. Or something... I never was sure the script made it all that clear.

If blood is not re-supplied with adequate pressure, the functionality of the nephrons will soon be permanently lost. Waste will immediately collect and clog things up (think New York City during a sanitation strike).

The only alternative is a connection to a dialysis machine, which requires the kidneys to route the unfiltered blood outside the body for mechanical filtration and return. It may keep you alive, but it's

a real hassle. That's why people have kidneys removed and somebody else's kidneys transplanted.

Transplants always come with collateral issues. Best if the native kidneys take off again. If they remain inactive, potassium begins to collect (for some reason) and in sufficient quantity is always deadly. It must be eliminated. Minutes begin to count.

Chapter 10

July 26 a portion of Lynn's entry:

...[H]is kidneys have to start working or we have some tough decisions to make. My heart is broken and I'm so very sad. But still my hope is built on nothing less than Jesus' blood and righteousness. I dare not trust the sweetest frame but wholly lean on Jesus' name.

~~~~~~~~~~~~~~~~~~~

Other Voices

He looked bad, worse than anyone I had ever seen, and worse than he had before the surgery. He was completely out of it, unaware of his surroundings; he had a pasty complexion without color. Tubes and machines were everywhere, with background ICU sounds: Beeps, chirps, tones, whirring motors. The kidney specialist, Doctor C, and her nurse practitioner were there. They studied his labs, checked readouts, and held low discussions. Then they asked if I would speak to them outside the room. I followed, knowing what they would say.

Doctor C haltingly reminded me how very bad Curt's condition was. She told me his kidneys were shutting down, and that meant the beginning of the end. She waited for my response, and I asked if his death was now probable. She nodded yes; unless things changed, it was a near certainty. In tears, they both hugged me.

It was not a shock to me, as I had already come to that conclusion, but hearing it from the doctor was profound. I thought: How is one supposed to prepare for this? – Lynn

~~~~~~~~~~~~~~~~~~~

I knew nothing of this except a snatch of videotape in my head. Two white-coated technicians worked on a portable machine that emanated loud klaxon blasts (a submarine about to submerge, *Dive! Dive!*), followed by an obnoxious musical doorbell chime. The techs were frustrated because the machine was not working. I tried to tell them to call the factory rep – there is always a factory rep – but my voice would not work for some reason, so I went back to sleep despite the klaxon. I learned later that this was a malfunctioning dialysis unit, and I could not speak because of the tube down my throat.

*****

Nurse K resumed her debrief with me. "I was told your kidneys had shut down. A couple of the other cancer ward nurses visited you in CICU after your surgery, and you shooed them away, which was not like you. They reported that you looked terrible. There were machines all over you, tubes in and out, your kidneys weren't working, and your complexion was white and pasty. They had seen others like this in CICU and honestly did not think you would make it. We were all in shock; we couldn't believe it."

*****

In the CICU, post-surgery, I realized I was awake. Acoustic ceiling tiles came slowly into focus, there was a rectangular light fixture, and I heard low voices. I could not lift my head. My hands would not work.

Why could I not lift my head? Was that a restraint around it? Where were my hands? The brain commanded them to lift, but they would not.

Chapter 10

A face appeared... Lynn. She smiled and said something; I can't remember what. Probably, "Hi, welcome back," or the equivalent. My brother RC was in the room; I could hear his voice. He leaned over, and I could see his face. I tried to speak, but there was nothing there; no amount of work could produce a noise from my throat.

Eventually, I came to understand that I was intubated. The tube was down my throat; the natural reaction was raising my head and using my hands to yank away that horrible, intrusive obstruction. Hence the restraints.

It was the most helpless feeling of my life. But as I lay there, I tentatively rustled from side to side – no pain in the chest. Relief swept over me, and I began to suspect I might live through this. But I had no idea how close to the edge I remained, nor of the immense stress under which the nurses and staff were operating.

Eventually that day, my mind cleared, and I began to plan what must be done in my situation. Now, we all know, there was approximately *nothing* to be done except lie there and accept whatever multiple medicines were dripping into my arms. I think there were six simultaneous IV connections. My role was simply to breathe deep and try to survive the next 24 hours... so maybe my mind was, in fact, not all that clear after all.

But I needed communication. I was unreasonably seized with the need for a language that did not rely on audible words.

My brother was an electrical engineer and more. He was a ham radio operator, a retired Air Force officer and a veteran of many crises. I pointed to him with my left hand and flapped my thumb and fingers to indicate speaking. He got it immediately.

"You want to talk?" he asked.

I nodded and gestured for him to lean over the bed where I could see him. I knew I could not text because I could not see my fingers and did not believe I could generate an intelligible message on a cell phone keyboard. Morse Code was not practical because the dots and dashes have distinct lengths, very hard to duplicate without generating a tone, and we had no way to do that.

Several months earlier, I had read *The Tap Code* by U.S. Air Force Captain Carlyle Harris (Zondervan, 2019). The book described Harris' several years as a prisoner of war – held in what U.S. flyers called the Hanoi Hilton – after his F-105 Thunderchief had been shot down over North Vietnam in 1965. The tap code was a way to spell words one letter at a time with a pair of taps.

Imagine a five-by-five matrix of letters: A B C D E across the top line, F G H I J on the second line, and so forth. Leave out Q; use K as a substitute. Now you have a 25-character alphabet, five rows and five columns. Tap out which column you want (for example, three taps will be the column headed by C), and after a pause, tap the row you want (for example, two taps will be the second letter down, or H). This means *tap-tap-tap,* followed by *tap-tap,* represents H.

It is a tedious method, but I was sure RC knew of the tap code because he was a Vietnam veteran, his specialty was communication, and he was widely read. I was confident he had read everything he could about his Air Force brothers who had been held in captivity.

That morning in Cardiac ICU, Shelley, a close family friend, prayed us through this daunting communication dilemma. To Shelley, Lynn, RC and Mary, it was a heart-wrenching distraction, but they played along valiantly. For my part, I remained blissfully unaware of the cloud of death hanging over my bed.

Using modified hand signals, eye movement, head shakes and nods, false starts and guesses, and abortive attempts at writing on a pad I could not see with a pen I could not hold, it suddenly dawned on Lynn – prior to leukemia, I had bored her endlessly with the tale of the POWs – that I wanted to use the tap code.

RC scrounged a piece of paper and a marker and made the alphabet matrix for me, with the tap numbers for each letter, and then held it up in my limited field of vision. I could spell my name – barely – and we called it success. I collapsed, exhausted.

Around me, the vigil continued.

*****

Slowly, things began to improve. Enter Marva, and the power of prayer, once again. An excerpt from RC's Caring Bridge post on the evening of July 27 sums up the situation:

...[T]he medicine to stimulate the kidneys was administered this afternoon at about the same time Marva the marvelous appeared on the floor to do some housekeeping. Marva swung into the room and did some housecleaning of her own there with another of her Heaven-sent prayer sessions. We are attributing the kidneys starting to work to that prayer of hers, as much as the medicine... Overall, my assessment is that Curt is very tired but in no distress and all indications are that all the immediate concerns are under control...

Where would I be without Marva?

I think I know.

The kidneys gradually began to resume functioning, and after two days of dialysis, I returned to my room. Still unaware of the death watch that was held for me, I quipped to the nurses, "I had never thought that coming to the cancer ward would be an upgrade."

Theological Contemplations

Looking at it now, it was nonsensical, this driving desire to be able to communicate. But at some level, I think this is characteristic of all humans; we need social contact. *It is not good for man to be alone,* God said once upon a time in the Garden (*Genesis 2:18*).

A favorite Bible passage of many is Proverbs 29:18. *Where there is no revelation, people cast off restraint; but blessed is the one who heeds wisdom's instruction.*

I think the King James Version puts it better: *Where there is no vision, the people perish: but he that keepeth the law, happy is he.*

This has been applied (incorrectly, I believe) by many churches as an admonishment to develop a vision statement. I have nothing against vision statements, mission statements, or organizational planning (besides the fact that they lead to many rabbit trails and inconclusive grandiose proclamations). Still, I don't think this verse teaches it.

I think it just means we need to hear what God says. Without that, we can go through all the motions and find ourselves hitting only foul balls.

The revelation of God – the "vision" – refers to God speaking to the people. In Old Testament times, this was usually in the form of a prophet: *Thus saith the Lord!* When there was no communication, the people ran amok. By contrast, when there *was* communication, the people could understand His instruction – His "law" – and obey it to their happiness.

And a related thought: We also need to hear from one another. The Caring Bridge website asserts that *A quick comment, no matter the situation (positive or negative), can boost morale by 28.2%.* I'm not sure how they know that, but I can say this: Every comment posted on my CB site told me someone was watching and boosted my incentive to stay in the fight. I had this (perhaps warped) idea that having started the battle with my tough guy persona, I must not give up now.

Chapter 10

The Caring Bridge posse had made a considerable emotional and spiritual investment in my cancer. Capitulation on my part would cheat them out of the win they rightfully deserved. There were maybe 250 people following me, and I know many others ghosting: Reading, following, and praying without posting.

The leukemia may kill me – or, more likely, it would be a collateral agent, Doctor A's adamant defense notwithstanding – and that surely would be too bad. Still, there would be no dishonor if I stayed in the fight. Folding up, on the other hand... never.

There was the posse to consider.

Hanoi, North Vietnam, 1965

In the POW compound in the 1960s and 70s, the North Vietnamese guards never detected the tap code.

The American prisoners of war used it to tap the Lord's Prayer and the Pledge of Allegiance laboriously and faithfully from cell to cell, passing those precious words on to one another, one single memorized character at a time. This was their usual Sunday morning worship service.

And if you are an American, and can read that paragraph without emotion, you might want to review both documents and contemplate the price of freedom in your generation.

The tap code was delivered in various creative ways, not only through tapping but also through hand signals, coughing, spitting, sweeping with a broom, moving objects across the floor. One POW, when tasked to sweep the hallway, routinely swept out "Seek God here." He later died in captivity.

~~~~~~~~~~~~~~~~~~~

Other Voices

May 1972. I was Weapons System Operator in a McDonnell-Douglas F-4E Phantom II fighter when we were shot down near the Vietnamese DMZ (Demilitarized Zone) and immediately captured. I was held for ten months until released with all the POWs, 40 pounds lighter and with five different parasites. U.S. bombing in North Vietnam had been halted between 1968 and 1972; I was the 14th American shot down after the bombing resumed.

Contact between prisoners at Hoa Lo prison (the Hanoi Hilton) was strictly forbidden, yet the POWs found many ways to subvert this edict and communicate using the tap code and hand signals. The tap code can be tapped, swept (with a broom), visual (poke a straw through a tiny hole in the wall), or move a door or other object, coughing or spitting, clearing throat, etc.

Communication with others was absolutely essential in maintaining hope and fighting against despair – it kept alive the will to survive and made surmounting the daily challenges possible. – Captain, U.S. Air Force (name withheld)

~~~~~~~~~~~~~~~~~~~

John McCain, by the way, eventual U.S. Senator from Arizona, was interned in the Hanoi Hilton for over five years. Freedom was offered by virtue of his birth; his father was a serving U.S. Navy Admiral. The younger McCain, suffering from a shattered leg and two broken arms in a rough ejection from his stricken A-4 Skyhawk, accepted release only on condition that the other POWs be freed along with him. The request was denied. He remained captive, with injuries that permanently impaired him.

McCain's story is only one of many.

*****

Chapter 10

In CICU, we never used the tap code again. The next day, the tube was removed, and I could speak semi-intelligibly. Or at least croak meaningfully. I hope we will never need the tap code… but it will be there if we do. While this may now seem pointless, the morale boost I felt from having attempted and succeeded at a frankly impossible task was monumental.

There I was with Walt Whitman: *The knowledge of death on one side of me and the thought of death close by on the other.* Yet, like Whitman, fighting despair after the assassination of Abraham Lincoln, his "powerful, western fallen star," I began to feel a note of optimism, a breath of fresh life.

I had endured the catheter risk, the atrial fibrillation, and the ruptured spleen, any one of which could quite reasonably have killed me. I was not yet aware of the extent of the kidney failure I was experiencing then, and it would be weeks before I understood the nearness of that almost-killer. I began to think that perhaps I would survive after all.

Because I'm a tough guy, you see. Confidence returned there in the ICU.

Life was good; I was on the mend, the distractions were behind me, and soon we would return to the Main Event, which remained, after all, the Big L-word. I was anxious to get to the next level of chemotherapy.

But I had not reckoned with how slow one's body — specifically, the bowels — could be to recover from abdominal surgery. They were capable of displaying their displeasure by twisting themselves into knots — literal knots — seemingly worried about the trauma to their host, although it's anyone's guess how that could possibly benefit the host.

In the days to come, they would demand attention, and they knew how to get it.

Chapter 11

Caring Bridge Journal, July 30 – September 13, 2022

July 30
Update for Curt, 7pm [by Brudder RC]
Good recovery from splenectomy several days ago, kidneys started working after Marva prayed and the meds were changed (simultaneous events) so no dialysis needed (never mind those leg-inserted dialysis catheters that were installed, checked, then clogged before any dialysis could be done – those will be removed probably tonight). Blood numbers are looking very nice now, so bone marrow is working as we'd like it to. Legs still swollen, but earlier thinking was once the kidneys started working, legs would unswell (made up that word myself, rich language, English). But intestines are still not working, so that's the issue-de-jour, along with the chubby legs. Nose tube into stomach provides comfort whilst we wait on the intestines. As of this afternoon, the blockage is determined to be a physical twist in Curt's internal plumbing, said diagnosis divined by a radiologist based on the xray and CT scan yesterday evening. Praying for and waiting for an unprompted untwisting event, which we understand happens spontaneously sometimes. If no intestinal movement by tomorrow, then another CT scan with dye will be the diagnostic tool of choice to determine the path forward. In the meantime, no food or water (wait, isn't that prohibited by the Geneva Convention?). Egads. Curt's heart went into fibrillation for a few seconds today, the EKG team came up to the room (heart is monitored closely and continuously), ran an EKG and found no issues at all, PTL. Son Caleb Ross is in the room this evening with Curt, presumably to provide the barrier between Curt and any sustenance. Thanks so much to all of you for the continual prayers. James 5:16 "...pray one for another, that ye may be healed. The effectual fervent prayer of a righteous man availeth much." ---Brudder RC

July 31
Lynn's status report, hospital stay day 40
Curt had a good night last night, he slept well, got to sleep on his side for awhile (a big deal!) and his voice sounds better. That intubation tube did a number on his vocal cords but he was not as raspy this morning. Those are all very positive things.

Our big issue now is this blockage in his bowel. He's been without food or water for several days now, giving his bowel a chance to fix itself. It hasn't yet so they will do a CT scan with dye today. I don't know any of the possible outcomes from that since the doc came in at 4:00 am to talk to Curt about it. But here's something you can pray for; that Curt would start passing gas. That will be the first sign that things are working themselves out. Did you ever imagine that one day you would pray for flatulence? Me either.

Again, I wholeheartedly thank you all for holding Curt up in prayer. I am humbled by what you do for us. – Lynn

August 02

Chemo Day 39, hospital day 42. Abdominal surgery, such as the ruptured spleen last week, takes a long time to heal. Fluid continues to collect at the site and must be drained off. Right now that is an external mechanical drain; eventually the body can take care of it but the volume is overwhelming at present. Until the draining is under control, we can't really move forward with the Next Big Event, which is, oh yeah I forgot, the leukemia treatments.

Abdominal drainage control will be measured in days or weeks.

Meanwhile I am on a liquid diet... and you have no idea how good vegetable broth and cranapple juice tastes for breakfast. They are also tailoring a special drip diet with proteins etc.

Leukemia: We finished Induction Phase (first round of chemo) on Day 28. There are 4 months of Consolidation Phase yet to go: Chemo 1 week out of every 4. Onc Doc says when the body has recovered from the spleen thing we can start Consolidation, but I know he is anxious to start it soon as possible.

Romans 8:18 For I reckon that the sufferings of this present time are not worthy to be compared with the glory which shall be revealed in us.

Dinner is here! With jello this time! Curt

August 02

Chemo Day 39 suppl. Actually they doctored the jello with so much protein that it's the consistency of bearing grease. I choked it down but I think I have a case for false advertising.

Got up a couple of times today, sat in a chair for an hour or so working on... throughput.

Tonight they shot me up with magic juice and x-rayed it (or something) and determined there were no mechanical blockages. That's good news, but if you hear the term "barium enema" you might want to hide. Or take hostages.

Bedsores: I understand I have one started, and worked with an aide to develop preventive measures involving pillows and frequent repositioning.

Chapter 11

Prayer: for some reason I have been unable to sleep at night. I spend nights awake, then watch some PragerU or equivalent, and by 600am I am exhausted... and sleep through the morning doctor consults. Pray I could sleep at night.

Proverbs 3:24 When thou liest down, thou shalt not be afraid: yea, thou shalt lie down, and thy sleep shall be sweet. Curt

August 03
Lynn's status report, hospital stay day 43

Curt had a good night last night. Thanks for praying about that. You all are amazing and I'm so thankful for you all. It's so good to belong to this faithful support group. Much love to you all.

Curt is still weak tho he is getting stronger. This coming Monday was when the next part of the leukemia treatment was supposed to start, but I'm guessing that will be delayed. One thing I remember the oncologist saying was we have to treat with chemo again or the leukemia will come roaring back. I've asked so many times and I'm humbled by the fact that you all are so gracious to let me do so. But Curt needs to start getting stronger, start eating real food, and the, ahem, throughput as Curt called it needs to happen. He also needs to get strong enough to get off oxygen. He's better but still a long way to go. All that to say he needs to get better so the treatment for the real issue can begin again.

Gratefully, Lynn

August 17
2nd Chemo Day 7 (hospitalization 57). One of the doctors explained last night that the insurance holdup about the Cresemba and the Rydapt [medications] is that the hospital is already incurring the cost of those treatments, so the insurance company sees no reason to pick up the expense in their budget. Just let the hospital pay for it on an in-patient basis.

Now, I know you will say that at $8000 a day for the hospital room, and because both insurances are actually Medicare and come from the same fund, it makes no sense to fight with one another. But everyone has a budget and it is a little bit logical to push expense from my budget to your budget.

We shall see what develops.

And this just in this morning; Insurance has agreed to pay 75% of the monthly cost of Cresemba, which still leaves me with $1700 per month out of pocket, which is a non starter for me, given that I could remain in-patient and get it at no cost. So the hospital case worker is preparing an appeal to the drug manufacturer asking for it for free. That appeal will take a week or two, and those requests are frequently approved.

So I remain here for the time being.

Meanwhile, do not consider my 57 days in a state of the art medical facility with fresh water, nutritious meals, outstanding staff and working air conditioning a hardship. For perspective, consider what others have endured:

1943: Louis Zamperini ("Unbroken"), 47 days on a raft in the Pacific, then POW in Japan, 2-1/2 years.

1967: John McCain, held in Hanoi Hilton, 5-1/2 years

1979: 52 US diplomats held hostage in Tehran, 444 days.

1987: Baby Jessica, age 18 months, in a well in Midland Texas, 56 hours

2010: 33 men trapped in a mine in Chile, 69 days

Pray: Exercise, PT, witness to staff, Gods timing for discharge.

Romans 8:23-24 even we ourselves groan within ourselves, waiting for the adoption, to wit, the redemption of our body. 24 For we are saved by hope…

That we are, and hope abounds continually! Curt

August 20

2nd Chemo Day 10 (hospitalization 60). Lynn and I walked down to the cafeteria for some (hyper acidic) Starbucks and then sat in the shade on the front drive, see the selfie. Beautiful morning for it, almost but not quite as good as sitting on our own front porch.

Not much new, slept well, am being overseen by the charge nurse. She gets called a lot (a lot) by other nurses who need assistance, which leads me to believe the charge nurse is the overseer of patients who don't need much overseeing. I like her, she is extremely personable and competent, but I don't get to see her much.

Doctor this morning said NOT SO FAST on when you're going home… sure maybe Tuesday, but there remain insurance issues related to the home use of Cresemba, the Lion King anti-fungal.

So, as has been the case the last three times I was about to get out, we'll just take it a day at a time. I'm good with it.

Statler Brothers: Counting flowers on the wall, that dont bother me at all… Don't tell me I've nothing to do…

But I have been able to see a few old movies on YouTube: Audie Murphy westerns, Clark Gable and Burt Lancaster in Run Silent Run Deep, Dad's favorite The Dirty Dozen. Also I have gained a new appreciation for classical music; I highly recommend Bach's Brandenburg Concerto #6, third movement. I would say it is a piece filled with joy and exultation from start to finish, but that sort of comment might jeopardize my tough guy image.

Pray: Gods timing on discharge, diligence in PT, relationships with staff.

Roman's 8:25-26 But if we hope for that we see not, then do we with patience wait for it.26 Likewise the Spirit also helpeth our infirmities…

Chapter 11

Romans chapter 8 is worth memorizing if you have a mind to do so. I find KJV is easiest to memorize because the phraseology is so unusual and specific. The Word makes wise the simple and enlightens the eyes (Psalm 19).

Patience is good! It is a brother to endurance! Curt

August 25

2nd Chemo Day 15 (hospitalization 65). A bonus day, not only a shower this morning but a professional massage also. St Francis offers a free massage to inmates every 30 days and it is delightful. The masseuse identifies herself as the Knot Nazi, and it is an appropriate appellation.

Cresemba was denied again, so now I must write a letter explaining my financial situation and asking them to reconsider again. Which I shall do. It will take them a day or so to pass judgment, and if they actually approve they will ship the product direct to our home address. It must be received there prior to release from the hospital in order to ensure continuity of care. Which means probably end of next week for discharge. If they reject again it could be longer.

☺ whatever. The Chaplin assumes I am really frustrated but I explained to her, The more you treat it like a sitcom, the easier it is.

Judges 8:4 And Gideon came to Jordan, and passed over, he, and the three hundred men that were with him, faint, yet pursuing them.

Faint, yet pursuing! That's us! Curt

September 07

3rd Chemo Day 2 (hospitalization 78). I am not exactly "running the stairs" but I can do half a dozen reps up and down a flight of 10 steps without using the handrails. Can't say I like it, or that my respiration is normal when I finish, but it's some degree of success in regaining the animal-like conditioning I would like to say that I had prior to this development.

And then, as if sensing I needed special care, Quinn the Therapy Puppy came to visit. He is a golden retriever in English Cream color, I am told. He is quite well behaved and was intensely interested in my tennis shoes. Nice visit!

And now: The hospitalist laid out the new discharge plan: They will send me home this Saturday after the first 5 days of this chemo. The balance of this treatment I will do out-patient at home with oral meds, which will include Rydapt and Cresemba. I will be left to my own resourcefulness to find a way to pay for the drugs. Besides those two there are a myriad others, mostly generic (and mostly free).

After this round, the next two chemo treatments will be entirely out-patient, with daily trips to the clinic for a 2-hour IV drip.

So the plan is to be discharged on Saturday 10 Sep.

That may actually happen, and if so I'm looking forward to it. I might miss some of the cafeteria food, however.

And the people. Certainly the people.

2 Corinthians 5:4 For we that are in this tabernacle do groan, being burdened: not for that we would be unclothed, but clothed upon, that mortality might be swallowed up of life.

We'll see how it works! It's an adventure! Curt

September 13

HOME AT LAST!

After 83 days in captivity we were evicted to the free and scary outdoors. We came home at 5:00 pm yesterday. This is much like moving out of the dorm at the end of semester... many small bags of toothpaste, phone chargers, pens and pencils, yada yada.

And a substantial bucket of drugs along with a packet of paperwork akin to buying a car.

The nurse corps formed up for us by the elevator to say goodbye and we ran the cheering gauntlet. They are indeed a noisy and ebullient lot.

It was a pleasant evening, so for the first time in 3 months we had crackers and cheese on the deck with Lynn's brother Ross.

I am poignantly aware that without the well wishes and prayer support of you all in the Caring Bridge Brigade this outcome would have been significantly different. An integral component of the fellowship of the saints is that we may bear one another's burdens. There are those among you who have performed yeoman's service in this regard, without which I am quite sure one of us would not be making this particular journal entry. You have buoyed my spirits enormously and given me a reason to stay in the fight. To say I am deeply appreciative is a considerable understatement.

There is still a ways to go: I am finishing this round of chemo at home (ergo the pills) and will do two more sessions of outpatient chemo in October and November. Interspersed are multiple clinic visits including IV work, blood tests, injections, consultations etc.

Each chemo session has its own set of side effects, potentially ranging from mouth sores to nausea to... other nasty eventuations. Those effects have been very light so far. May they remain so.

For the next two months, no lifting, no dusty environments, lots of walking but no excessive exercise. Driving is probably okay. So there.

With this entry I will bring the daily posts to an end. Look for updates on Fridays going forward. If there is something special, however, I will post it.

I cannot tell you how grateful I am, and how humbling it is, to have you all following this saga.

Okay... enough syrupy monologue.

Pray: Pills - there are a lot to keep track of, and in quantity they can be nauseous. Protection - the white blood cell count will not be truly normal, Lord willing, until March or April, until which time I am highly vulnerable to infection. Productivity- meanwhile I have all this unemployed mental capacity (such as it is) which needs to remain occupied. I have some thoughts about that.

James 5:16 ...pray one for another, that ye may be healed. The effectual fervent prayer of a righteous man availeth much.

Don't I know it! Glad to be home! Curt

Inflection Point 6 – Bowels and Bureaucracy

~~~~~~~~~~~~~~~~~~~

Other Voices

Today's CB journal [August 25] *blew me away. Once again, the medicine was denied! Another setback! Countless days in the hospital. The "main event" that never goes away – Curt has cancer. So, I texted him affirming how he is putting shoe-leather to the Biblical response to suffering: Hanging in there, not losing heart or quitting. What an INSPIRING GIFT he is to me – demonstrating what a healthy, manly Biblical response to potential disaster looks like.*

I told Curt that the tiny "☺ whatever" in his post today spoke a book full to me! He has a surrendered heart to whatever comes along, even if it's incredibly difficult or frustrating. – Ron

~~~~~~~~~~~~~~~~~~~

I will deal with this delicately, but I think you can understand what I mean by throughput. What goes into a man, said Jesus, will not defile a man because it eventually passes out of his body *(Mark 7:18).*

While I am sure the Great Physician understood bowel blockage, I don't think the New Testament ever records Him dealing with it. Just as well: I'd rather try to decipher the inscrutable and all too frequent instances of demon possession in the Gospels than be faced with plain language about... throughput.

The bowels do not take well to abdominal surgery. This comment was made in passing by a surgeon a few days after the splenectomy. *(Now you tell me!)* The intestines seem to object to their territory being invaded, and they develop a reluctance to cooperate in the daily production of... throughput.

So, they don't. Instead, to halt this production mid-flow, as it were, they constrict, twist, convulse and generally make a significant nuisance of themselves like a petulant three-year-old who refuses to unlock the front door for you when you have retrieved the newspaper on a snowy morning in your jammies.

But in this case, of course, we are discussing the *back* door.

Three days after the surgery – long enough for the problem to become evident and for the tough guy patient to begin to whine for a solution – the doctor raised the possibility of a barium enema.

Johns Hopkins (hopkinsmedicine.org): Barium is a dry, white, chalky, powder that is mixed with water to make barium liquid. Barium is an X-ray absorber and appears white on X-ray film. **When instilled via the rectum,** *barium coats the inside wall of the large intestine. This allows for visualization of the inner wall lining, as well as the size, shape, contour, and patency* [obstructions] *of the colon. (Emphasis added.)*

That phrase about something being "instilled via the rectum" does not bode well.

The barium brew shows the professionals what the intestines look like. It was vital for them to understand the extent of the blockage, one explained to me, for in extreme cases, there could be a colon rupture. This is a perforated bowel, allowing contents of the colon to be spilled into an unsuspecting abdomen, which is as bad as it sounds. It ranks right up there with a ruptured spleen. Scary terms like peritonitis and septic shock are used in this context. I was told painkillers might not be effective, and there was a high likelihood of death. But first, there would be a few days of unspeakable agony.

I wanted no part of it. *Bring on the barium brew!*

I will not describe the procedure in the enema lab in detail because it's too graphically gritty, but it is unpleasant for the patient. Not quite like a chest full of broken glass, but unpleasant, nonetheless.

When it was done, I lay on the transport gurney, gasping and exhausted with after-shock. A doctor told me, "This is not an official read-out on your results, but I can tell you we found no major blockages. There were some twists and kinks, and I believe the introduction of the barium solution itself probably straightened all those out." He paused. "You may have found it difficult to go Number Two before this."

With breath still labored, I nodded. "That's why I'm here."

"Now," he said, "I think you will find it difficult *not* to go Number Two for a few days."

He was right, but I will also not describe that development in detail other than to comment that the nurse assistants in the cancer ward are *troopers. Seriously!*

On the cart, rolling my way out of the enema lab, I asked the transport driver girl to pause. I spoke, still haltingly, to the four technicians who had operated the machine and were now cleaning everything up, including mopping the floor. I sensed a great deal of splashy cleanup was usually required after one of these procedures.

"Thank you all for doing this," I said. "I cannot imagine that when you were in grade school, you decided to administer enemas for a living, but I want to thank you for choosing this career path. Apparently, somebody has to do this, so I thank you much."

One replied, "We are glad to do it for you, sir. And thank you for your sincere comments. We rarely get to hear that from anyone."

I'll bet he was right. Sincere cursing perhaps, but appreciation, probably not so much.

As a footnote, RC asked what it was like. I replied that as a gesture of my brotherly love for him, I would purchase a barium enema for him for Christmas, and he could experience it for himself.

~~~~~~~~~~~~~~~~~~~~
Other Voices

Several years ago, I had served as pastor of Curt's church. When I heard of his leukemia, I decided to visit him in the hospital. During the meeting, I found that Curt was humbly aware of how God was caring for his every need through each unexpected and often unwelcome turn of events. This was not a surprise; I would not have expected anything else at this most challenging moment in his life.

Curt demonstrated faith, with an awareness of how to see Jesus – rather than evil – while walking through the valley of the shadow of death. Although I came to his room to minister to him, it was he who lifted my spirits on that special Sunday afternoon. – Rob
~~~~~~~~~~~~~~~~~~~~

Speaking of the gut and lower tract, which subject I know you and I would both like to leave ASAP, there was yet another development in the War on Curtis delaying our return to the Leukemia Campaign. This new thing showed up some three days after I was back on 7-North, and all those nurses so glad to see me began to re-think the welcome.

Chapter 11

Having nothing to do with the bowel blockage and the barium enema (which I decided was my new best friend in terms of treatments), I developed a bacteria called C. diff. Centers for Disease Control (cdc.gov) says the proper name is *Clostridiodes difficile*; it is an infection that causes diarrhea and colitis, the latter being an inflammation of the colon.

The back door is getting a lot of press here.

Even better, not only does C. diff create... unpredictable and untimely throughput-ish activity... it is also highly contagious. *Do tell.*

The risk factors for C. diff, again per the CDC, are (a) being age 65+, (b) being in the hospital, and (c) being treated for cancer. *Yes, we have a winner!* And, not to make sport of a malady that takes itself very seriously, one in 11 C. diff patients will die, even under controlled hospital ward conditions.

I had been threatened with statistics so much that it hardly made a dent by this time. *So what?*

One of the doctors explained that we all have natural flora growing in our gut all the time. This organic process breaks food down into nutrients and is a normal part of the digestive system. If the process is stopped, it must be restarted. C. diff attacks that process and must be treated promptly to avoid long-term complications.

Think of this like yeast in a starter lump of sourdough bread. In bygone times, before IGA and Hy-Vee and Kroger and Piggly Wiggly, the starter lump was a routine wedding present for the new bride to help set up her household. Without the starter lump, you don't make bread.

The hard part for the hospital staff is the protocol for treating the C. diff patient. Any nurse, doctor, aide, cafeteria runner, flower deliverer, counselor, etc. who interacts with multiple patients runs the risk of unwittingly carrying a contagious disease from one room to another during their shift.

When a visitor comes to see me, they see me and leave the ward; no risk of taking anything next door. But after the nurse comes to see me, she moves to the next room.

For this reason, all the staff must tediously gown up each and every time before they enter my room. Uncomfortable, unstylish, and unbreathable plastic ghillie suits are conveniently provided on a cart in the hallway; they must glove up and don the near-full coverage suit before entering my room, and then discard it on the way out. This routine is needed for ten days, the recommended treatment period for C. diff.

This makes one unpopular with the nursing corps.

Lynn found the solution to unpopularity, however. It involved the daily delivery of a small fortune in donuts, sweet rolls, or other carbohydrate-rich delicacies to the nurse station. It didn't make the ghillie suit routine any better, but they seemed to look forward to her daily arrival. The C. diff protocol is a fact of life in the cancer ward.

After a few days of IV antibiotics, C. diff went away. So while there was a seemingly interminable requirement to continue treatment with an oral med, I had no more trouble with it.

~~~~~~~~~~~~~~~~~~~~
Other Voices

I was settling into bed for the night when my mom came to my room and told me that Mr. Curt had leukemia. That day, and many others, I prayed to the Lord that He would save Mr. Curt and heal him. Even though I was worried and scared, I knew that the Lord would fulfill His plan for this situation. Finally, he is getting better, and the Lord has strengthened my faith more than I ever thought was possible. – Cora, age 14

~~~~~~~~~~~~~~~~~~~~

And then began the Battle of Insurance Coverage. At this point, I had been inpatient for almost two months, and once the C. diff protocol played out, there would be no reason for me to remain. The chemotherapy Consolidation phase could be done outpatient, with occasional trips to various clinics for IV drips, lab work, and doctor consultations.

The limiting factor came down to the cost of the medication.

Under Medicare rules, a hospital is reimbursed a monetary amount for every inpatient with cancer; this may take the form of a lump-sum payment plus a small daily reimbursement. Usually, this is vastly inadequate to cover the hospital's actual cost of care. It is based on an average expected length of stay. If a hypothetical patient – call him Poindexter – is released in fewer days, the hospital wins and keeps the extra money. The hospital goes in the hole if Poindexter is high maintenance and requires a more extended stay. Too bad for the hospital, but Poindexter's level of care is unaffected by this, which is the point of the system.

The hospital does not get a vote in this arrangement. The reimbursement amounts are announced, and they are expected to go along. Unlike the United Methodist Church's connectional system, there is no provision to buy your way out.

Because of logistical constraints, outpatient Consolidation chemotherapy requires oral meds rather than IV drips. All those bags of highly regulated fluids, so easy to handle in a hospital environment by certified staff, must be converted to prescription pills for uneducated boobs like Poindexter to manage at home. If Poindexter is lucky enough to have stumbled into a very rare form of AML – such as the FLT-3 variant – the capsule form of the drug can be expensive.

And it gets better. Because FLT-3 was only recognized formally by the Food and Drug Administration less than five years before Poindexter's diagnosis, the still-patented drug treatment has minimal availability. Supply and demand being inviolable rules of the universe, it amounts to $1,500 per chemo cycle.

And it gets better still. Because of the dreaded Fusarium fungus, which may also afflict poor Poindexter, a daily dose of an anti-fungal is required. There is a reasonably low-cost treatment, but it does not play well with the new and exotic FLT-3 drug, which requires its own unique (and new, and still-patented and expensive) anti-fungal drug. *Of course, it does.* Unfortunately, it also has limited availability and costs around $6,800 per chemo cycle.

In my case, remarkably similar to Poindexter's, I would require six cycles of Consolidation chemotherapy.

Originally, Doctor N had advised that after the Induction phase there would be four Consolidation cycles of chemo. Later, however, he recommended extending this by two additional cycles. Most patients, he explained, find the side effects of chemo treatments overwhelming; they are worn out and discouraged after four months, but he considered that duration a minimum to ensure the AML remains at bay. The more cycles of chemo, the better; each cycle, he believed, would push the cancer away for an unknown period: A month, a year, a decade.

The doctor pointed out that I had experienced virtually no side effects, and he deemed that I could easily withstand the two additional treatments. I have no idea why I was thus favored – beyond, of course, my right living and clever wit. (Or maybe not so much.) It comes out the way it comes out.

So, the good news was I could increase the mostly uncertain effectiveness of the chemo cycles by 50%. The bad news was I could increase the highly certain cost of the chemo cycles by 50%. Besides the other 11 required daily pharmaceuticals (almost free by comparison), I was facing $8,300 per month, times six months, or $49,800 in treatments.

I was expected to see this as a happy development.

While my insurance would reduce those costs, it would not reduce them enough to make them palatable.

Chapter 11

Perhaps it should go without saying, but I had leukemia, was out of work, and could not earn an income because of a significantly compromised immune system. (*Maybe I should write a book*. The thought crossed my mind.)

As with any of us, daily household expenses continued; bills for electricity, gas, water, telephone, internet, cable TV, insurance premiums, and property taxes continued unabated. The additional financial burden of the outpatient meds was a non-starter for me. I explained this to C, the very competent hospital case worker assigned to me.

To C's credit, she represented my case well with the administration. She was pleasant and understanding – and had instructions to evict me at the earliest possible moment.

If I remained inpatient, the hospital was obligated by law to provide all the meds, effectively at no charge, not to mention the daily rate for the room and cafeteria service. While a bill was rendered, it was written off to the wholly inadequate Medicare reimbursement. Too bad for them, but I couldn't fight every battle.

Caseworker C initiated requests to my Medicare Advantage provider, asking for greater coverage for outpatient meds. When that proved ineffective, she pursued grant programs to reduce costs. Finally, she approached the pharmaceutical providers directly, asking for assistance on my behalf.

All this took weeks, submitting applications, being rejected, appealing the rejections, having the appeals rejected, reviewing the rejections of the appeals, and resubmitting to different funding sources. Meanwhile, Doctor N was anxious to get on with the treatment. Waiting too long between Induction and Consolidation was a sure way to have a resurgence of leukemia. We would lose all the ground we had gained, which would harm the doctor's reputation – never mind how Poindexter and I might fare. We had already run too much time off the clock with minor distractions like a-fib, a burst spleen, non-functioning kidneys, and a lower tract on strike.

After the spleen episode, during the C. diff treatment, Doctor N called on a Wednesday morning, grudgingly wearing the required plastic hazmat suit. I elevated my electric bed to a sitting position to converse with him. I asked him if I could call Lynn, who would want to hear the conversation; and when he agreed, I put her on speaker.

"I am aware of the financial constraints of outpatient treatment," he began, "but we must get on with the Consolidation phase of your chemotherapy. So here is what we will do." He shifted in his chair. "We will dismiss you tomorrow to give you a few days at home. Then on Monday, we will ask you to return to the hospital and check in again. We will administer the week of chemo on an inpatient basis. That way," he concluded, "the hospital will pick up the charges for your treatments until we can find a lower-cost method."

Doctor N was not an insurance guy. A superb oncologist, to be sure, but lacking in an appreciation for the vagaries of Modern American Medical Compensation, which some might see as Socialism by Alternate Nomenclature. As it happened, I had an ace card of which he was unaware.

When I began employment at age 65 with the small meat processing sales outfit, my boss was 28 years old. His last name happened to be on the side of the building, so at least he had that going for him. In addition, he had a friend of approximately the same age who was breaking into the insurance game. Running a small family-owned business, the boss could ask every employee to meet with his buddy for individual discussions once a year to review insurance needs. In other words, a mandatory sales pitch.

I'm sure they could be excused if someone objected, and the boss, who actually demonstrated a high degree of integrity, would certainly not hold it against them.

I went to the appointment as a new employee. I decided to buy the cancer protection policy (through the modern miracle of payroll deduction) because I wanted to be nice to the well-spoken young man making the pitch. I had no thought that it would ever be needed. Similar to other reimbursement policies, this one does not pay the healthcare provider. I had Medicare for that; but instead, it simply pays cash compensation to the individual for being sick. Most insurance carriers offer similar policies.

This type of insurance is offered to compensate for out-of-pocket expenses which continue to arise during an extended hospital stay. In that way, it acts like a disability income policy.

As soon as I received the initial cancer diagnosis, I became intensely interested in the heretofore ignored but quite generous benefits package.

Have I mentioned that I love America?

Like most on the market, this policy paid a cash benefit for each day of hospitalization. For the first 30 days, they would pay a flat daily rate. Beginning Day 31 of continuous hospitalization, the rate doubled. The higher level would be paid until discharged; when readmitted, the daily benefit would reset to the original rate. It is important to note that this is paid directly to the patient, not the hospital.

At the time of my conversation with Doctor N, I had been in for 48 days, and I could do the arithmetic in my head. Each day I awoke to the "ka-ching" of a virtual cash register in my imagination. And now... here was the doctor suggesting that I be discharged, only to return four days later. I could feel the marginal revenue slipping away as I studied his ill-fitting blue gown.

The doubled daily benefit – now in jeopardy – amounted to income that would replace most of what I had lost by not working. Tax-free.

The doctor wasn't nuts, merely uninformed. But I felt the need to steer a path to avoid a down-and-dirty discussion of personal finances. As Dan Dailey once said to James Cagney, "Think fast, Cap'n Flagg!" *(What Price Glory, 1952)*

"So, doctor," I began conversationally, "I very much appreciate your consideration of my situation. That is enormously helpful." I showed my appreciation with my most sincere smile. "But why are you sending me home?"

There was a pause, during which I retained the fixed smile and tried not to show that I was holding my breath.

He examined his fingernails. "Most patients in your situation," he said tentatively, "after spending so much time in the hospital, need the psychological adjustment of going home for a few days. They need the time to relax in more comfortable and familiar surroundings before beginning the ordeal of chemotherapy."

He was unaccustomed to being challenged, which put him a little off his game. This was somewhat out of his wheelhouse. This was not medicine; this was patient psychology.

In four decades of business-to-business sales, I had seen this scenario scores of times. When the other party deviated from his primary area of expertise, he floundered and needed a lifeline. Such was now the case with the good doctor. I, on the other hand, suddenly found myself on my home turf.

"Doctor," I said, and he made eye contact with me. I held his eyes for a beat, then deliberately enunciated the question. "Do I look to you like a guy who needs psychological adjustment?" I emphasized the last two words just enough to show faint disdain.

His eyes suddenly came alive. "Do you mean you do not want to go home first?"

"Doctor," I said, with a firm shake of my head. "Please do not send me home. If you send me home, I will have to call in some of the boys to rearrange the furniture in the living room. I'll have to decide which bedroom to use and which bathroom I can access. I'll have to get a walker. I'll have to get home health care for physical therapy. And then, in less than a week, I'll have to come back here." I wagged my head and frowned furiously at the enormity of the problems. "Just keep me here and start the chemo."

"You don't need the downtime?" he asked eagerly. But he had already turned the corner.

"Ask my wife," I said. "She will tell you. I am the same difficult person now that I was two months ago when I first showed up here."

Across the cell phone connection, Lynn laughed. She knew what was afoot. "That's right, Doc," she said. "He hasn't changed a bit. Besides that," she added, "the sooner you can start the chemo, the sooner we can get him out of there!"

"Wait here!" Doctor N said with excitement. "I am going to revise the plan!" With that, he fled from the room, ripping the hated ghillie suit away and stuffing it into a trash can.

Thirty seconds later, a nurse stuck her head in the door. "Curt!" she said. "Those pills I put on your table! Don't take them yet! We are changing the treatment plan."

Lynn: "Are we alone?"

"For the moment," I replied, "yes."

Quietly: "I guess it worked, huh?" She giggled.

"So far, so good," I said. "Thanks for your help."

"Anytime," she replied. Then, "I'm out," and she ended the call.

Theological Contemplations

I will never be persuaded that the human body came about by anything other than intelligent design. While I grasp only a fragile veneer of the science, I have seen first-hand the intricate complexities at work to keep a human functioning effectively. Few of us are excited to contemplate the visceral aspects of "throughput." Still, some sage has pointed out that regardless of astonishing technological advances, we will always and forever need plumbers in our midst.

Without apology, we can say with the Psalmist, *I am fearfully and wonderfully made; marvelous are Thy works, and that my soul knoweth right well. (Psalm 139:14 KJV)*

Like anything else medical, the introduction of the barium enema does little but assist the body in fixing itself. Others have pointed out that a surgeon's contribution mostly removes offending material so the body can reconstitute itself. The entire point of chemotherapy treatment, both the Induction phase and Consolidation phase, is to kill off the damaged white cells. The hope is that the bone marrow can then create new and healthy ones unimpeded.

A friend of mine has experienced minor internal bleeding for five years. He has been hospitalized off and on while doctors attempt to locate the source of the problem.

At one point, he underwent abdominal surgery where most of his intestinal tract was closely examined, inch by inch, spread out and looped over hangers above the surgical table (reminding the nurse who observed this of the gambrel known to deer hunters) before being re-inserted into his belly cavity. She told my buddy, the patient, about this incredible scene, and he later asked the surgeon, "How do you remember where it's all supposed to go when you put it back?"

"Oh, it's not as hard as you would think," the doctor casually responded. "You stuff it back inside, grab the edges of the skin and give it a few shakes. It all settles into place."

*****

Beyond medicine, there are constraints on money and resources in this modern world. I have always been intrigued by that story Jesus told of the shrewd money manager accused of mismanagement. He unilaterally reduced the debts of clients who owed his master. Jesus did not condemn but instead commended him: *Use worldly wealth to gain friends for yourselves, so that when it is gone, you will be welcomed into eternal dwellings. (Luke 16:9)*

I fear my reaction might have been the opposite, which would have missed the point entirely. The parable's teaching seems to be that we should hold this world's goods as mere tools; use them, says Jesus, to facilitate your acceptance by the final Judge.

If riches can be used this way, so can medical technology or any other application of technology. It is not a stretch to conclude that taking advantage of scientific advances can promote the kingdom of God. The trick is to refuse the inappropriate pride that accompanies the fitness of the body, the gathering of wealth, or the accumulation of gadgets. *(The lust of the flesh, the lust of the eyes, and the pride of life... 1 John 2:16)*

Besides this, it seems that the takeaways from profound life experiences should be reviewed, refined, and verbalized. What good has it done if we fail to internalize the learning and put it into practice? Like the accumulation and disbursement of money, it was only suitable for the moment. The opportunity to invest it for more lasting rewards will evaporate.

Guam, 1945

It was rare to see an actual Naval officer venture to the far end of the airstrip where the fuel depot lived. But there he was, roaring up in a Jeep, a real live lieutenant with a sour, determined look.

After a quick exchange of salutes, the lieutenant demanded, "Chief, are your men putting Navy gas in Army aircraft?"

Chief Petty Officer Ghormley was not exactly a political creature, but he understood a loaded question when he heard one.

All sorts of aircraft made their way to the Navy landing strip at Guam. When combat operations were underway, it was not uncommon to see a desperate pilot wrestle his stricken plane to any available safe landing spot. Anything was better than ditching in a shark-infested ocean. Frequently they needed emergency repairs; they always required fuel, and the fighters required ammunition. In many cases, the need was urgent as they had to return to the battle.

One could argue that the only reason for any American to be 10,000 miles from home in the South Pacific in 1945 was to engage in combat operations. The sooner the combat was over, the sooner they could all go home. The sooner a plane – any plane, Army or Navy – could be refueled, the sooner the combat would be over.

Unless the chief had missed something important, the point was to get it over with and go home.

But the Navy had its regulations, and woe be to the lowly NCO who disregarded them, even if he shared a last name with an Admiral.

"Oh no, Sir," declared the chief with a straight face. "You will never find these men putting Navy gas in Army aircraft." *You will never find these men...* Word choice is critical when responding to an officer.

"Well," said the lieutenant with a scowl, "you'd better never let me catch your men putting Navy gas in Army aircraft!"

Chapter 11

"Oh, no, Sir, you will never catch us putting Navy gas in Army aircraft! Sir!"

"Very well, then, chief," the lieutenant said, suspicious but mollified. "Carry on!" The gears ground and the Jeep roared away as it had come.

Dad watched him leave, shaking his head slowly in amazement.

Bureaucracy is a remarkable thing.

Whether the bureaucracy of insurance, the bewildering threat of killing disease, or the unexpected side trips into unwelcome and deadly complications, the lessons of the Journey into Leukemia have been the substance of this book. We shall see what fruit they can bear.

Let's close it out.

Chapter 12

Lessons Learned

I was discharged from the Cancer Center at Ascension St. Francis Hospital on September 12, 2022 – Day 83 of inpatient treatment. I had been wearing street clothes for two weeks, walking the halls daily, venturing outside for fresh air, and flirting circumspectly and harmlessly with nurses young enough to be my grandchildren. I was marking time until the second round of chemotherapy was concluded and the insurance issues were resolved.

The only complaint I had, which no one at the hospital seemed to take seriously, was that they would not give me a swipe card to access the nurse's squad room where the coffee pot was. This meant I had to continue to act nicely, and politely ask a nurse to let me in for my coffee. And refills.

One of the nurse assistants, exaggerating her African-American dialect, offered a tongue-in-cheek complaint: *Laud-o'-mercy, Curt, yo' still here?? If'n yo' can walk that good, yo' can walk good enuf to carry these here blankets fo' me!*

Through insurance concessions and grants, the financial impact of outpatient drugs was clobbered down to an acceptable level. The resulting charges were merely painful rather than life-altering.

As I contemplated the previous three months, I attempted to crystallize the conclusions I had drawn from the experience. Leukemia was a game-changer for me, as a significant medical issue is for anyone. I was determined not to let the occasion go by without extracting something valuable from it – something, that is, beyond another five or 15 years of living the dream.

Still using the laptop from work, although I was off the payroll and needed to give it back – I figured they would ask for it if they wanted it – I began to identify the lessons and universalize them. I wanted them to be relevant beyond the immediate application of fighting Acute Myeloid Leukemia.

Here they are in list form. I'm sure this is incomplete, clumsy, and inelegant – I have chemo brain, after all – but that fits right in with everything else I've done.

1.   *Optimism is infectious, genuine or not.* I was determined to make journal posts every day on Caring Bridge. Furthermore, the posts would be upbeat, light-hearted, perhaps a little sarcastic, cavalier, and humorous. Many days, I did not feel like posting (and I completely missed two days in CICU), but I gutted it out. The point is that while I could acknowledge real problems, I wanted to show that I intended to meet them. From reviewing the hundreds of comments on CB, many in the posse were strengthened and encouraged by this. Everybody loves a winner, even if he goes down in defeat. (Think Mel Gibson's character in *Braveheart, 1995.)* It's a contradiction.

2.   *Encouragement incentivizes success.* Every comment I received, whether on CB, text or email, phone call or visit, made me aware that a great cloud of witnesses was rooting for me. Once having gone public with the tough-guy approach, I found I could not back down. Maybe it's just the pride of life, of which the Apostle John speaks so condemningly, but I could not bring myself to contemplate retreat before the watching eyes of those who supported me. They deserved better, and I found myself buckling down to deliver a win to them.

3.   *Prayer is not our last resort but our first.* I get mightily tired of the dramatic refrain, often voiced in movies by the hero's friends who see him rise to the final challenge, "All we can do now is pray!" I think: *Hey, you jack-wagon, if you had tried that first, maybe your buddy wouldn't be in such trouble now!* (But that may not draw box-office success.) As I have probably made clear, I am not a seeker of modern-day miracles. But, on the other hand, I can see reality. The mouth sores, the ampho-terrible chills and the kidney failure were all turned around when effective, fervent prayer was applied by righteous people. Would those problems have gotten fixed anyway? Who knows? This is not a lab experiment; it's real life. As the label on the paint can says, *For best results, follow the directions.*

4.   *The more you treat it like a sitcom, the easier it is.* Once you get past Walt Whitman's *knowledge of death on one side of me and the thought of death close by on the other,* some of the developments were downright laughable. From the loss of the grocery store job in high school to the evil boss who wanted to fire me but couldn't, to the kidney failure after a busted spleen *(What else can possibly go wrong??),* the acknowledgment that one has so very little control over these externalities is an immensely freeing concept. Be faithful, be cheerful, accept reality, and watch it go by. Moses was told, *Stand firm and you will see the deliverance [of] the Lord... Exodus 14:13-14.*

5.   *Don't suffer in silence, and also don't suffer in public.* Paul urges the church, *Carry each other's burdens, and in this way you will fulfill the law of Christ (Galatians 6:2).* It takes two parties to do this, one to admit the burden and the other to help carry it. I cannot be a practical part of the church unless I am willing to talk about my burden; others cannot be an effective church without helping to carry it. But no one wants to be discouraged, disillusioned, saddened or depressed by my burden's gruesome or tedious details. Instead, the sharing must be upbeat, brief, and optimistic, even in tragedy. This may be hard to pull off, but it keeps the posse in the game.

6.   *Never let a crisis go to waste.* This saying has been around a long time and was popularized by Rahm Emanuel, Chief of Staff in the first Obama Administration, more recently, Mayor of Chicago (one of the few not in federal prison) and U.S. Ambassador to Japan. Political conservatives widely panned his statement as indecorous cynicism. Which was true, of course, but be that as it may, it reveals a nugget of truth. A personal crisis surprises us, but it does not surprise God and is a Heaven-sent opportunity for developing maturity and – dare I say – toughness. *James 1:2 Consider it pure joy, my brothers and sisters, whenever you face trials of many kinds, because you know that the testing of your faith produces perseverance.*

7.   *A hard trail is not the same as a closed trail.* Sometimes guidance comes to us as doors are opened or closed, but the open/closed status is not often clear, and it is up to us to discern the difference. Sound counsel from a trusted source can help with this. Grit and determination are sometimes required to make the journey, whether in school, business, child-rearing, marriage... or cancer. There is no profit without stress. One thing I have observed: The trails seem only to get harder, not easier.

8.   *We do not always get to choose the trials we face; only how we face them.* Imagine the shock and dismay when the window of Paul Tibbets' B-17 was blown out on his first bombing mission, or when the Navy Chief found Marines stranded on a Pacific island reef under fire, or when the 17-year-old sailor found himself under attack on the very first day of his war, or when the ER doc said matter-of-factly, "That's leukemia." We should never be paralyzed into inactivity by surprise; leave that to the deer in the headlights. As the John Wayne poster says, "Life is tough; it's tougher if you're stupid." This is a good argument for anticipating Bad Things That Might Happen and planning accordingly. It's why we have fire extinguishers in the house.

Chapter 12

In the above list, the last one is last because it best summarizes my understanding of this battle with cancer: *We do not always get to choose the trials we face; only how we face them.* I don't know if I could have verbalized this before the diagnosis. It only became clear as I progressed through that long and tedious experience. Facing up to trials is a matter of mindset, decided ahead of time, applied in actual situations, and burnished with experience. Isaiah 50:7 is applicable here: *Because the Sovereign Lord helps me, I will not be disgraced. Therefore have I set my face like flint, and I know I will not be put to shame.*

*****

I asked one of the nurses whether working in the cancer ward was a different experience than the other floors of the hospital. "Oh, I'd much rather work here in oncology," she said. "In the other assignments, you find lots of self-inflicted pain, mostly drug and alcohol-related problems. There, it's more common to find bitterness and anger or resentment. Some patients are mean to the nurses; they take it out on us. Here, the population is entirely different."

"How so?" I asked, intrigued.

"Well, look at the type of patient we have. You are all generally older and have a more mature perspective on life. And the big thing," she smiled, "is that everyone here was taken by surprise. Nobody ever expects cancer. It's not your fault; there is no blame associated with it. And," she added, "I suppose because you guys are all older" – this nurse was a young 20-something – "you tend to see cancer as a problem to be solved instead of something to be ashamed of." She smiled again; I could tell she was glad to have this conversation.

"There is more optimism here," she concluded, "and it's rare that a patient treats the nurse disrespectfully."

*****

Reflecting on this journey, I recognize that there were six inflection points (not counting the original diagnosis) — those incidents where life was on a knife edge: The initial two-week life span projection, catheter insertion, atrial fibrillation, ruptured spleen, kidney shutdown, barium enema. (The ruptured spleen hurt the most; *wowser.*)

I cannot overstate the value of the posse — the Caring Bridge Brigade — in this journey, and I am humbled each time I think of them. I cannot imagine the isolation and despair of going through this alone. As they beseeched God in prayer, these saints not only delivered me from the mouth sores, the ampho-terrible chills, and the kidney failure — these I can enumerate easily — but probably also accounted for landing on the right side of the knife edge. All that, plus the fact that I never experienced any of the much-promised side effects from chemotherapy.

Your mileage may vary. No one makes promises about this sort of thing, or believable promises, at any rate. Some people suffer terribly from cancers, and many die, and it's probably not because they are bad people or have bad friends who don't pray for them. It comes out the way it comes out. *We do not always get to choose the trials we face; only how we face them.*

So, am I a tough guy? Like each of us, I have been through toughening experiences all my life. But sometimes, it is as challenging to tease out the lesson, think it through, and draw conclusions valid for the next battle as it was to go through the trial in the first place. I think I have figured out that succeeding against whatever wicked thing comes my way next requires reflecting on the wicked thing that came my way last.

In this story, I have sought to point the way for the one who faces an insurmountable challenge. We must find a way to remain perched on top of the circumstance rather than being crushed under its weight.

And this "tough guy" thing, I believe, boils down to three distinct, sound principles, embodied so succinctly in 2 Timothy 1:7, which passage made an appearance in Chapter 1. *For the Spirit God gave us does not make us timid, but gives us power, love and self-discipline.*

- Power is strength under control.
- Love flows through us to serve others.
- Self-discipline acknowledges the reality of a challenge and rises to meet it.

None of these three makes the slightest accommodation for timidity, and neither should we.

Toughness does not reject Christian maturity but instead demonstrates it. Possessing strength (mental, spiritual, or physical) while keeping it under control is a testimony not to oneself but to the One Who is served. That strength ought to be seized and employed the way it was intended: To be a channel of God's grace to others. Strength is revealed when one is self-disciplined to acknowledge a challenge and show the determination to meet it.

May God grant us the courage to show forth His power, love, and discipline while we may.

So yeah, I'm a tough guy, or at least a work in progress. And I can hardly wait for the Next Challenge That Will Surely Come. *I'm ready. Bring on the alligators.*

Afterword

After I was out of the hospital, Derek called and asked when we could have coffee. I invited him over. My immune system was highly compromised, and he had lots of young kids at home, so we sat on my back deck, far enough away from one another that he probably wouldn't kill me with some infection or other. I made sure he was downwind.

Derek sold real estate, was half my age, and had a habit of asking insightful questions that suggested he was genuinely interested in learning how to manage his life and career.

Once we settled on the deck with coffee, he asked, "Now that you're 'Old Curt' and retired" (*and almost dead, he graciously did not add*), "what advice could you have given 'Young Curt' when he first began his career?"

It was a good question. I had thought about this issue and had already organized a response.

I launched into a short soliloquy; there were three discrete ideas.

First, develop and maintain your political contacts. I had the privilege of meeting many high-quality and accomplished people during my career, both at work and in outside activities. I had met some through our kids' school and others through business clubs, church, and other situations. These were not all whom one might think of as the great and powerful – although some were – but they each had unique value. My life and career would have been more prosperous had I taken the time to develop stronger relationships with them. Some could have helped me later as I navigated a life of work; others would have enriched the experience. All would have added value.

Second, see to your own needs. I have gone into this in some detail earlier, but it is a component of a practical, profitable life not to be overlooked. One should never confuse self-interest with selfishness, a self-absorbed and self-defeating focus on one's own interests to the exclusion of others. Instead, it acknowledges that God has equipped one with gifts to be exercised for His glory. So, exercise the skills, don't apologize, be profitable, and don't try to fix everyone else's problems. Instead, give others the grace and the space to make their own way.

Third, don't take yourself too seriously. Passion for a chosen pursuit is a good thing, but taking it to extremes can become so tedious that no one wants to be around you. In the emergency communications business, I associated with "true believers," those practitioners who put such a high value on a fast and accurate emergency response that nothing else seemed as important as delivering a first responder to the scene in record time. A quick response is excellent and should never be understated or compromised... but other components of the total response picture are also important: Competent treatment, specialized training, the right supplies and equipment, and a budget that balances costs with capabilities. A single-minded focus is good until it blinds one to effectiveness.

Those three concepts may not be the secret to life, but they help make the rough places a little smoother.

Acknowledgments

I honestly don't know where you would find a more dedicated, competent, knowledgeable, considerate, and attentive staff than at the Cancer Center at Ascension St. Francis Hospital in Wichita, Kansas. I looked forward to the daily visits from doctors and their associates, not only for their treatment capability and genuine interest but because they were also highly entertaining. The doctors were determined not to lose me, despite my tendency to stumble into one deadly medical disaster after another: "Not on my watch!" one proclaimed.

The nurses, assistants, and staff: When I'm in trouble, I want this cadre on my side. An unruly lot, they are absolute troopers, and words cannot do justice to my appreciation for them. They are pleasant, upbeat, communicative, tender, business-like when required, and damn-the-torpedoes aggressive in an emergency. I owe them my life. Thank you, thank you, and thank you. They also like donuts.

Jeffrey Schiesser, Information Technologist Extraordinaire, was of enormous help in facilitating the Caring Bridge interface, my website, and the technical details of blogging, audio recording, and other hands-on dark techo-arts. Russ Womack guided this novice would-be writer through editing and proofreading with full engagement, sincere interest, and awe-inspiring attention to detail. Professional illustrator C.S. Fritz designed the cover for this book and effortlessly created the cover art out of thin air… a skill I can only view with wonder. I think it's quite catchy!

Many thanks to Mike Andrus, former pastor and current friend, for the kind Foreword. He is a rare and brilliant man of God who thinks clearly, speaks simply, and loves deeply.

Ross Schoneboom, Lynn's brother, supervised our three dogs every day for three months while Lynn spent time with me at the hospital. Hounds gotta eat. For this, Ross was unpaid, but we did invite him over for dinner once, by way of thank you. I would hate to offend him by offering actual compensation.

And the Caring Bridge Brigade: You took seriously the Apostle's admonition to "bear one another's burdens," and you bore mine with over-the-top dedication and sincere prayer. There are warriors in your midst.

The hospital housekeeper Marva, whose heaven-rocking prayer sessions demolished medical obstacles, was used by the Lord in a most powerful way to bear witness to His mercy toward a frail cancer victim, who's passing the world would barely have noticed. Her commitment to the God of the Bible and the power of prayer was a testimony to all of us who observed her, and no doubt makes serious spiritual waves among the staff and patients at St. Francis.

Besides Marva, there were actual chaplains at St. Francis, notable among them Chaplain Kristin Gilmore, who frequently looked in on me or found me in a hallway during my many excursions. Her interest was genuine, her prayers sincere, and her visits greatly encouraging.

My wife Lynn, whose reward for her work is having to put up with me for yet another season, took this disaster in stride with loving attention and determined focus. Her detailed notetaking of doctor visits, consultations, medications, and procedures corrected most of my chemo-brain recollections of what happened and when. Plus, she also saved my life that night in ICU... there is that.

About the Author

Curt Ghormley lives with his wife Lynn in Benton, Kansas, a small town outside Wichita. He holds a Bachelor of Arts degree from the University of Kansas and an MBA from Wichita State University.

In 2022, Curt's world was turned upside down with an unexpected diagnosis of Acute Myeloid Leukemia (AML), a fast-moving cancer that kills 12,000 Americans each year. Doctors also identified a rare genetic mutation of white blood cells, the dreaded FLT-3 variant, that cuts the five-year chance of survival to less than 15 percent. Curt spent 83 days in the hospital with multiple life-threatening complications, but still managed to post a social media journal update every day, except for his time in the Intensive Care Unit.

After retiring from a successful career as a communications technology sales manager with a Fortune 500 company, he was suddenly plunged into the fight of his life. By God's grace, he has survived it – so far – with his trademark optimism, resiliency, and humor.

Curt and Lynn have two sons. Both boys completed college degrees and served stints in the U.S. Army, spending some harrowing time down-range in distant dusty places, and thankfully coming back in one piece. They are both married and gainfully employed in the private sector. There are three grandchildren.

Curt's hobbies are reading, woodworking, welding, four-wheeling, shooting, and playing the tuba.

Learn more about him at www.alligatorpublishing.com.

Made in United States
Orlando, FL
28 May 2023

33582320R00143